CANCER REPORT

The Latest Research
How Thousands are Achieving Permanent Recoveries

An Instruction Manual Including:

Patients Personal Recovery Guide
Comprehensive Support & Resource Directory
Inspirational Success Stories
Worksheet Pages for Personal Notes

Contributions by:

W. Douglas Brodie, MD ◆ Susan Silberstein, PhD
Candace Pert, PhD ◆ Lawrence LeShan, PhD
Lydia Temoshok, PhD ◆ Greg Anderson
Andy Bernay-Roman, RN, MS, LMHC ◆ Hippocrates Health Institute
Optimum Health Institute ◆ Ryke Geerd Hamer, MD

By
John R. Voell
Cynthia A. Chatfield

CANCER REPORT

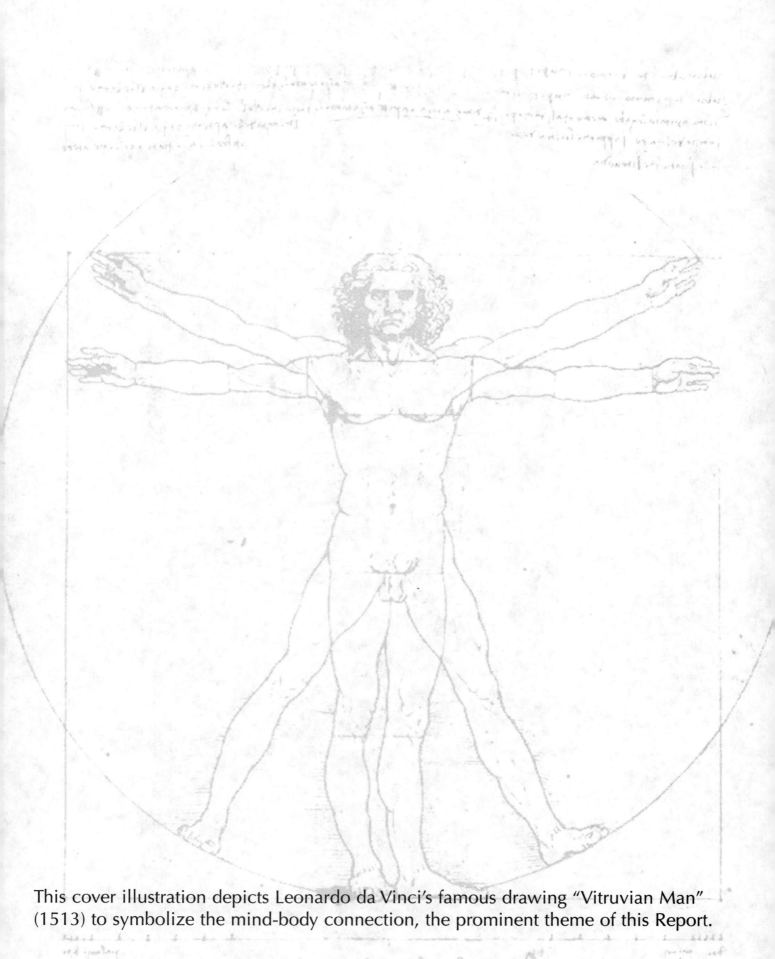

This cover illustration depicts Leonardo da Vinci's famous drawing "Vitruvian Man" (1513) to symbolize the mind-body connection, the prominent theme of this Report.

CANCER REPORT

The Latest Research
How Thousands are Achieving Permanent Recoveries

An Instruction Manual Including:
Patients Personal Recovery Guide
Comprehensive Support & Resource Directory
Inspirational Success Stories
Worksheet Pages for Personal Notes

Contributions by:
W. Douglas Brodie, MD ◆ Susan Silberstein, PhD
Candace Pert, PhD ◆ Lawrence LeShan, PhD
Lydia Temoshok, PhD ◆ Greg Anderson
Andy Bernay-Roman, RN, MS, LMHC ◆ Hippocrates Health Institute
Optimum Health Institute ◆ Ryke Geerd Hamer, MD

By
John R. Voell
Cynthia A. Chatfield

Cancer Report

Disclaimer: This Report should not be regarded as a
guide to self-diagnosis or self-treatment. The cooperation
of a qualified healthcare professional is essential if you choose
to apply the principles and techniques discussed in this book.

Editors—Lee Marmon
Tamsen Fox

Layout & Cover Designs—Tamsen Fox

Library of Congress Control Number
2 0 0 5 9 0 4 3 8 2

ISBN 978-0-9768770-0-4

Change Your World Press
PO Box 9211
Naples, FL 34101

www.cancer-report.com
Printed in the USA
on acid-free paper

DEDICATIONS

In loving memory of Arlene, Joey, and Peggy.
~John R. Voell

For Tom, who inspired it all.
~Cynthia A. Chatfield

CONTENTS

Preface   xiii

Acknowledgements   xvii

Introduction   1

PART I   *Scientific Research & Case Studies*

Chapter 1   **Why You Should Read CANCER REPORT**   27

Chapter 2   **A Modern Integrative Cancer Practice:**
               W. Douglas Brodie, MD   31

Chapter 3   **The Success of Mind-Body Therapy:**
               Susan Silberstein, PhD   51

Chapter 4   **A Cure for Cancer:**
               Ryke Geerd Hamer, MD   79

Chapter 5   **Cancer as a Turning Point:**
               Lawrence LeShan, PhD   103

Chapter 6   **The Scientific Connection**
               Between Emotions and Health:
               Candace Pert, PhD   119

Chapter 7   **Do You Have a Cancer Personality:**
               Lydia Temoshok, PhD   145

Chapter 8   **Creating Recovery:**
               Optimum Health Insitute   161

Chapter 9   **A Life-Changing Boot Camp:**
               Hippocrates Health Institute   171

Chapter 10 **Jump-Start Your Healing:**
Andy Bernay-Roman, RN, MS, LMHC   **185**

Chapter 11 **Your Can Be a Cancer Conqueror:**
Greg Anderson   **199**

PART II *Patient Action Plan & Resource Directory*

Chapter 12 **A Formula for Healing**   **233**

Chapter 13 **Patients Personal Recovery Guide**   **239**

Chapter 14 **Comprehensive Support & Resource Directory**   **307**

PREFACE

About the Authors

John's Story

I have dedicated the last seventeen years to cancer research and authored several publications on the subjects of cancer and health.

The *Cancer Report* is the latest of my publications on natural health care. My motivation and passion to do the research for this came from the loss of my dear friend Joey to a brain tumor, my son's mother to lymphoma, and then a close friend, Peggy, to breast cancer.

This Report is profound in content, delivering an essential message to save lives and prevent the needless physical, emotional, and economic suffering of individuals and families. I say this not because of my role in this work... but because of irrefutable research contributed to this Report by so many talented, dedicated professionals.

The potential social and economic value of this Report could be measured some day in millions helped and billions saved.

Here is a little more about my background leading up to the *Cancer Report*.

Although I have an MBA in Marketing and regard myself as an experienced and astute businessman, I like to tell clients that I have a self-awarded PhD in natural/holistic health from the last thirty years of study, research, and "real life" experiences. During this time I have passionately pursued my education and research in this field as an author, counselor, and holistic practitioner.

I have instructed hundreds of students in thirty-five states and four countries in natural health and healing. I earned a Natural Health Certificate from the A.R.E.

Medical Clinic and studied and spent many years working with the medical intuitive/psychologist Ross Peterson.

In 1998, I authored the lifetime reference guide and tape series: *The Ultimate Prescription: How to Create Physical, Emotional & Spiritual Health!* This program was inspired by the work of my dear friend Ross Peterson. Peterson was a gifted visionary who was the source of the insights in this guide. For almost thirty years, Ross was also my psychologist and advisor.

As one of the three co-founders of the Natural Awakenings Publishing Corporation in 1999, I have worn many "hats" and have marketed, motivated, mediated, and meditated. This position has put me in touch with all the cutting-edge natural health treatments and therapies. The corporation's magazine of the same name now has the largest circulation in the natural health field.

In closing, I just want to say, I know all about being seriously ill. I have personally been able to heal my kidneys, gall bladder, stomach ulcers, a hiatal hernia, diverticulosis, as well as chronic lower back problems without the "pills" of conventional medicine or surgery. I was also able to overcome depression and substance abuse.

It is our greatest hope to be able to help you and your loved ones.

You are fortunate, indeed, to possess a copy of this Report.
We have done our part....
Now it is up to you to do yours.

Cynthia's Story

When my friend John Voell approached me with his passionate plea to assist him in creating this Report, I said "Yes—absolutely!"

I have spent the last fifteen years learning and working within the fields of alternative medicine, holistic education, and spirituality, after being inspired and guided to this path by the death of my life partner in 1990 from metastatic colon cancer. Tom was diagnosed at age thirty-eight and given just four months to live; yet he was able to survive four full years beyond this grim prognosis. I attribute this to his unabashed joy in life even in the most difficult of circumstances, to his determination to create more time to be with his children, and yes—to the amazing gift of love that we shared during those years.

At one point, Tom achieved a complete remission with no sign of disease anywhere in his body, yet the cancer returned with a vengeance within six months. If he and I had known then what I now know about cancer and healing, I believe that he would still be here. I now think that Tom's cancer eventually returned because he did not understand the need to identify and address the repressed emotions of a lifetime, including some long-held angers and resentments. I wish I could go back in time and offer him the information contained in this Report. Several years after his passing, my dear Mother suffered the indignities, pain, and invasive procedures of conventional cancer treatment, and experienced one of the most difficult and horrifying deaths imaginable. I knew then there must be another way.

I later joined the newly founded National Foundation for Alternative Medicine (NFAM) in Washington, DC, and spent the next four years learning firsthand about dozens of holistic cancer treatments and protocols used internationally. As the Vice-President of Educational Services, I interacted with hundreds of cancer patients who contacted NFAM for help and I was able to offer these patients vital information via personal conversations, seminars, and clinic reports. More importantly—I was able to offer inspiration and hope. I want to reach and help many other patients and their families through the powerful and life-altering information contained within this Report.

John and I want to offer an understanding of the reasons why illness may develop, without creating a sense of guilt. We want to empower patients to take responsibility for their own healing, to educate them about how and where to begin, and then encourage them to take action to create their own healing miracle. If you have cancer, there is some inspirational and profound information in this Report that will make you think long and hard about how you got to this place in your life—and what kind of joyful and fulfilling future you want to create as a survivor.

And please remember—*there is always hope.*

ACKNOWLEDGEMENTS

We want to thank everyone who has been involved in this project by inspiration, contribution, and example. We want to extend special appreciation to Mary Voell Jones, Dr. Susan Silberstein, John Voell III, and Susan Q Wood for their invaluable guidance and assistance in bringing the *Cancer Report* to life.

This space is provided for your personal and/or support group notes.
PLEASE immediately record your ideas, insights, and inspirations as they occur to you.

_____

_____

_____

_____

_____

_____

_____

_____

_____

_____

_____

_____

_____

_____

_____

_____

_____

_____

_____

_____

_____

_____

INTRODUCTION

Please imagine the following scenario... which may be all too familiar to some of you:

You are "in remission" or receiving powerful drugs.... You painfully recall the previous six months... your body wracked with cancer... the tenth chemotherapy treatment after your surgery... your body feels completely alien to you because of the radiation.... You have spent most of your life's savings on invasive treatments that made you feel worse than before... they barely numbed the pain... the treatment has aggravated your anxiety... and the prognosis is still gloomy.

You have no idea why you have this cancer... you do not smoke... you have no known exposure to environmental carcinogenic agents... but you have had great stress in your life.... You wonder, in both times of lucidity and intermittent bouts of hazy consciousness, is there another way?

This *Cancer Report* is an emphatic YES that proves there is another way. This Report was written to show how thousands are achieving complete recoveries from most forms of cancer. This research reveals how these cancers can be arrested as well as cured through mind-body healing.

Because this material presents hard scientific data and clinical reports, the Report may be crucial to your life and your recovery. These cancer survivors, scientists, and healthcare professionals have all reached the same conclusion: you can have a complete and permanent recovery by addressing and removing emotional issues.

Organization and Substance of the *Cancer Report*

The *Cancer Report* is co-authored by long-time associates John Voell and Cynthia Chatfield. John has long believed that despite the many publications in this field, there was still a need for one text bringing together many healthcare professionals to make the cumulative case for mind-body cancer treatments. The *Cancer Report* is so significant because it presents in one single work a variety of experts who all—separately—make essentially the same fact-finding determinations. The *Cancer Report* is divided into two comprehensive parts.

This space is provided for your personal and/or support group notes.
PLEASE immediately record your ideas, insights, and inspirations as they occur to you.

Part I (contributing professionals and case studies) presents detailed examinations of the work of eminent and pioneering researchers in the field of mind-body medicine, innovative institutions providing holistic treatment facilities, compelling summaries of case work, and remarkable individual success stories of cancer conquerors. If available, relevant contact information has been included so the reader can directly access work and services offered by the contributors.

The chapter subjects included in Part I were selected in a variety of ways. There were many outstanding potential candidates for this Report and those chosen reflect a representative sample. Some were known to John through his extensive cancer research and some to Cynthia from her work at the National Foundation for Alternative Medicine. Some contributors were personally interviewed and additional research was derived from numerous websites and publications.

There is a cross-section of researchers, including medical doctors, scientists, psychotherapists, cancer survivors, other healthcare professionals, and holistic institutes. All are highly regarded in their respective fields and offer a collective impact. You will note that there is much "first person" commentary. Although there is a narrative structure, we have chosen to have the contributors speak in their own voices as much as possible.

While the information in each chapter is similar in message, each reveals special insights from different backgrounds to give you a wide spectrum of evidence. You begin with the story of an extraordinary medical doctor and end with an ordinary man sharing his extraordinary insights that led him to conquer cancer. Like a symphony in many parts, you will experience the harmonious convergent movements of the subsequent chapters that build to a crescendo... the incontrovertible confirmation that you have the power to remove the underlying psychological causes of your cancer.

Part II (action plan and support/resources) enables you to incorporate this knowledge into your own daily routine by providing an easy to use step-by-step Patients Personal Recovery Guide. The Report concludes with comprehensive resource listings that cover nearly every conceivable necessity of the many and varied personal needs of most cancer patients. This directory, based on years of research, has been carefully put together and can be employed with great benefit by not only cancer survivors but also their families, friends, and personal healthcare providers.

This space is provided for your personal and/or support group notes.
PLEASE immediately record your ideas, insights, and inspirations as they occur to you.

For the convenience of the reader, worksheet pages are incorporated facing every page of text. We want you to personalize this Report by immediately recording your thoughts and ideas that can support your recovery.

Concepts and Terms

The idea of cancer and conventional cancer treatment has a long history in our culture. For example, the first hospital specifically for cancer patients in the United States was established in 1904. The well-known National Cancer Institute, the American Cancer Society, and the Institute for Cancer Research are just three of the many organizations and research foundations devoted to treating and eliminating this frightening disease that has grown to such epidemic proportions.

Government research and private organizations have long existed to administer cancer treatments (including surgery, radiation, chemotherapy and other drug regimens). These are the "conventional" methods of treating cancer that are familiar to us all. Conventional medicine is practiced by medical doctors or doctors of osteopathy and by their allied health professionals, such as physical therapists and registered nurses. Other terms for conventional medicine include allopathy, Western, mainstream, orthodox, and traditional medicine. But these options are not the only paradigms available and, as we sadly know, they have failed far too many cancer patients.

There is a growing movement to perceive effective cancer treatment in ways quite different from exclusive reliance on these traditional techniques. These newer methods have been described as being "holistic," "complementary," and "alternative." Holistic refers to treating the whole person and causes. Complementary and alternative medicine (CAM) "is a group of diverse medical and healthcare systems, practices, and products that are not presently considered to be part of conventional medicine" (this definition supplied by the National Center for Complementary and Alternative Medicine). Complementary medicine is used together with conventional medicine. Alternative medicine is used in place of the more standard practice. Some conventional medical practitioners are also CAM health providers. The latest term used to describe combining alternative methods with the conventional ones is "integrative."

This space is provided for your personal and/or support group notes.
PLEASE immediately record your ideas, insights, and inspirations as they occur to you.

This Report focuses specifically on mind-body medical connections and the role of emotions in causing and eliminating cancer. An inclusive word is the new science of "Psychoneuroimmunology" (PNI). This term can be defined by its constituent parts:

> Psyche—the mind component or study of psychology, the cognitive and emotional processes involving mood states.

> Neuro—the neurologic connections (e.g., neurotransmitters and neuroendocrine secretions), or the study of neurology.

> Immunology—how the immune system (e.g., the cellular components) is impacted, or the study of immunology.

One suggested working definition of PNI is an interdisciplinary science that studies the interrelationship between psychological, behavioral, and neuroendocrine processes and immunology.

An Overview of the Development of Mind-Body Science

[Some of the following section is abstracted and revised from the article "Psychoneuroimmunology" by Jay Quinlan, found on the International Medical and Dental Hypnotherapy Association (IMDHA) website, in the second series, article #54 at: www.infinityinst.com/article_index.html.]

The name "Psychoneuroimmunology" was introduced in 1975 by Dr. Robert Ader, director of the division of behavioral and psychosocial medicine at the University of Rochester in New York. Dr. Ader believes that there is a link between what we think (our state of mind) and our health and our ability to heal ourselves. A study conducted by his research team showed it is possible to condition the immune system to connect communication through mental processes. The autonomic nerve system can suppress immunity through a conditioned mental response to chemotherapy, even in its absence. Returning patients to some feeling of control over their circumstances may create a positive outlook and attitude.

Psychoneuroimmunology, then, is the scientific field of study investigating the link between bi-directional communications among the nervous system, the endocrine (hormone) system, as well as the immune system, and the implications of these linkages for physical health.

7

This space is provided for your personal and/or support group notes.
PLEASE immediately record your ideas, insights, and inspirations as they occur to you.

A Brief History of Mind-Body Medicine
[Some of this material provided courtesy of Susan Silberstein, PhD]

It is interesting how cultural history has affected medical philosophies, high-lighting the dichotomy between Eastern and Western medical beliefs, and ultimately returning to the holism that provides the foundations of this Report. For millennia, traditional Chinese medicine has claimed that the organs of the body reflect various mental or emotional conditions.

Throughout the history of Western culture there has been much controversy over the mind and body connection. Many ancient medical belief systems asserted that the mind and the body should be treated as one. As far back as 400 BC, the great philosopher Socrates taught that "there is no illness of the body apart from the mind." The Classical Greek philosopher and "Father of Western Medicine" Hippocrates cautioned against limiting the range of healing possibilities. He believed that health is a state of harmony within the self and between the self and one's environment. For Hippocrates, whatever happens in the mind affects what happens in the body.

Centuries later, in the Middle Ages, a twelfth century Hebreo-Spanish physician, Moses Maimonides, wrote: "The physician should not treat the disease but the patient who is suffering from it." In the sixteenth century, German physician Paracelsus, the "Father of Pharmacology," used the power of dreams and visualizations as adjuncts to his medical treatments, and wrote about their influence in a healing process that involved body, mind, and spirit.

In contrast, contemporary Western physicians usually only inquire about the symptoms of the ailment and then prescribe a particular medicine. This system is derived from the seventeenth century philosophy of Rene Descartes of France. He believed "there are two distinct and separate substances in the world: matter, which behaves according to physical laws; and spirit, which is dimensionless and immaterial." Thus mind and body were treated as totally separate entities. The Cartesian philosophy brought an extremely mechanistic approach to medicine with the theory of a specific etiology, that is, every disease or infection is caused by one specific micro-organism. Western culture thus accepted that pathogens were the cause of all disease. This is a linear disease concept with a limited objective more aimed at absence of symptoms than achieving biological balance or optimal wellness.

This space is provided for your personal and/or support group notes.
PLEASE immediately record your ideas, insights, and inspirations as they occur to you.

The dichotomy between mind and body largely governed medicine for two centuries, at which point another dramatic change of direction took place. Neurologist Jean Martin Charcot became fascinated with the healing powers of the mind in the nineteenth century. He observed that under hypnosis mental patients suffering from hysterical paralysis could stand and walk. This laid the groundwork for the theory that chronic emotional problems can develop into physical ones; that is, emotions not expressed in words or actions find expression in physical ailments. One of Charcot's students, Sigmund Freud, carried his teacher's work further in suggesting that physical symptoms are related to past repressed traumatic experience.

In 1909, British physician Sir William Osler, the "Father of Modern Medicine," observed: "The care of tuberculosis depends more on what the patient has in his head than what he has in his chest." Ten years later, this concept was validated by Dr. Tohru Ishigami of Osaka, Japan, in a scientific report on the "Influence of Psychic Acts on the Progress of Pulmonary Tuberculosis." Ishigami concluded that the key to disease progression lay in the "emotional life of the patient," including failure in business, lack of family harmony, jealousy, nervousness, and death of a loved one.

Dr. Walter Cannon, a professor of physiology at Harvard University studied the need for mental and physical balance. In 1935 he coined the term "homeostasis," the body's self-maintaining inner state of harmony. He believed all of the body's related physiological processes could be affected by stressful life experiences, fatigue, and worry.

Hans Selye, prominent endocrinologist of McGill University in Montreal, carried on Cannon's work and experimented with animals, placing them under different adverse physical and mental conditions. He noted that in certain situations the body consistently adapted to heal and recover. These studies validated that emotional attitudes affect physiological states. Selye researched the impact of stress throughout his lengthy career and published *Stress Without Distress* in the 1970's.

By the mid 1970's with Harvard University leading the way, Psychoneuroimmunology began emerging as a serious scientific discipline. Over the last twenty-five years, the field of PNI has truly come into its own with a vast array of research studies. All of this work confirms that the next frontier is that of the human mind and that the potential of the mind for healing the body is virtually limitless.

This space is provided for your personal and/or support group notes.
PLEASE immediately record your ideas, insights, and inspirations as they occur to you.

Current Research in the Field

It was once thought that the brain sent out information substances to respond to the various problems in the body and that this communication was a one-way direction. But now we know that the central nervous system virtually controls the body's defense mechanisms.

EVERY THOUGHT, EMOTION, IDEA, OR BELIEF HAS A NEUROCHEMICAL CONSEQUENCE.

These natural chemical messengers, called neuropeptides, were originally assumed to be found in the brain alone. Pioneering research by neuropharmacologist Candace Pert revealed that these neuropeptides are present on both the cell walls of the brain and in the immune system. Pert's research contributions are described in a later chapter of this Report.

Recent research has indicated that an inextricable chemical link exists between our emotions (including all stress in our lives, both good and bad) and the regulatory systems of the endocrine and immune systems transmitted through the central nervous system. These studies emphasize the importance of expressing our emotions both verbally and physically in appropriate and effective ways.

There are a multitude of mind-body therapies and the application of this field is truly cross-disciplinary. Many techniques are used by a variety of professionals: medical doctors, nurses, naturopaths, osteopaths, energy body workers, practitioners of Chinese medicine, and chiropractors for the body model; psychiatrists, psychologists, psychotherapists, social workers, hypnotherapists, and counselors for the mind model. Some of the techniques include:

Guided Imagery

Guided Imagery (or visualization) is a process involving the use of mental symbols to represent the changes the individual desires to happen. Patients are often encouraged to relax and imagine a journey described by the practitioner. This procedure may include visualizing that their problem is comparable to

This space is provided for your personal and/or support group notes.
PLEASE immediately record your ideas, insights, and inspirations as they occur to you.

many other things that they know to be true and curable. An example would be the body's ability to send the appropriate healing to a cut on the hand. No thought is required for this to happen, as it occurs naturally. While visualization has been used for many centuries, it gained a lot of attention in the 1970's when cancer patients were encouraged to use it to fight cancer cells. A good example of this approach can be found in *Getting Well Again* by radiation oncologist O. Carl Simonton.

Biofeedback

The word "biofeedback" was coined in the late 1960's to describe laboratory procedures used to train experimental research subjects to alter brain activity, blood pressure, heart rate, and other bodily functions that are not normally controlled voluntarily. The most common forms of biofeedback are electromyographic (EMG) and the electrodermal (EDR) sensors. These sensors allow persons to monitor their own muscle relaxation, heart rate, breathing patterns, and perspiration while concentrating on changing these patterns through visual or auditory cues given by the equipment.

Extensive research has demonstrated that biofeedback can help in the treatment of many diseases and painful conditions through relaxation. Most scientists believe that relaxation is a key component in biofeedback treatment of many disorders, particularly those conditions induced or aggravated by stress.

Hypnotherapy or Therapeutic Hypnosis

The use of hypnosis to assist individuals in their own healing is an old concept. Mesmerism is a therapy derived from the 18th century work of Franz Anton Mesmer. A 19th century British doctor, James Braid, named this sleep-like state "hypnosis" (from the Greek "hypno" meaning "to sleep"). Today the conventional medical community sometimes uses hypnosis but more often this technique is practiced by specialized hypnotherapists in the field of complementary medicine. Amazing results can be achieved with some patients, i.e. painless operations are possible without anesthetics by simply suggesting to the hypnotized subject that he will feel no pain. This is clearly another demonstration of the power of the mind to affect the physical body.

This space is provided for your personal and/or support group notes.
PLEASE immediately record your ideas, insights, and inspirations as they occur to you.

Recent breakthroughs in Psychoneuroimmunology studies now give increasing evidence of the connection between mind-body communication and the role of hypnosis. There are as many different definitions of hypnosis as there are beliefs about how it works. "Guided Imagery" and "Biofeedback" are, of course, forms of hypnotherapy.

What PNI offers us is a blueprint of cellular and molecular communication between mind, body, and gene that takes hypnotherapy out of the realm of magic and into a psychological practical reality.

Meditation

Meditation is a mind-body technique in which we quiet the mind to keep it focused entirely in the present moment. Its practice is rooted in the traditions of most of the world's great religions. There are dozens of ways to meditate and reap physiological benefits; however, none has been more scientifically validated than the specific form known as Transcendental Meditation (TM). Over five hundred studies have been completed on the physiological, psychological and sociological effects of TM. Research has been conducted at 210 universities and institutions in twenty-seven countries, and articles on TM have now appeared in more than one hundred scientific journals.

It has been demonstrated that with daily practice of TM, significant stress relief is possible. This can be measured by physiological changes such as decreased cortisol (the major stress hormone), decreased muscle tension, normalization of blood pressure, increased autonomic stability, and increased electroencephalogram (EEG) coherence. Other benefits include less anxiety and depression, an improvement in post-traumatic stress syndrome, decreased hostility, increased family harmony and enhanced self-actualization.

Extensive studies conducted by health insurance companies have shown that with all age groups combined, those individuals practicing TM displayed 50% less in-patient and out-patient medical care utilization compared to the control groups. The hospitalization rate was decreased by 87% for heart disease patients and by 55% for those with cancer. Meditators over forty years old have approximately 70% fewer medical problems than others in their age group.

This space is provided for your personal and/or support group notes.
PLEASE immediately record your ideas, insights, and inspirations as they occur to you.

How are these results possible from a seemingly simple relaxation technique? According to Dr. William Weir, a consultant in infectious diseases at the Royal Free Hospital in London, "At a deeper level, Transcendental Meditation restores the innate balance of the physiology. When the mind and body can function properly, the natural intelligence within the body can function properly, strengthening the immune system and the other self-repair mechanisms that naturally protect against disease."

All of the modalities that utilize the science of Psychoneuroimmunology are non-invasive and enable patients to have some degree of mastery over their own health and welfare in a world where they often feel a loss of that very control in their own lives.

Academic Resources For PNI

PNI has spawned a vast array of scientific and technical literature. The most detailed account is the massive two-volume study (of more than 1,500 pages) by Robert Ader (who originated the term) and other contributors, simply titled *Psychoneuroimmunology* (now in its third edition). Although relatively new and controversial, PNI is well represented in scholarly works, international research centers, and professional organizations.

There are dozens of university research programs specializing in PNI. One prominent research facility is The Cousins Center for Psychoneuroimmunology at the University of California, Los Angeles. This program is dedicated to following in the tradition of its founder, the noted author Norman Cousins. He joined the university faculty in 1978 in a quest for proof that a patient's psychological approach to illness could have an effect on biological states and health. Cousins was particularly interested in the impact of positive emotions and attitudes: purpose, determination, love, hope, faith, will to live, and festivity. If the brain played an active role in the healing process, might it be consciously directed for that purpose?

Cousins believed that a good vehicle for making such discoveries was the emerging field of Psychoneuroimmunology. He appointed a task force of high-caliber scientists whose representation encompassed the breadth of the field. [The preceding information on The Cousin's Center is an edited abstract from the website: www.cousinspni.org/history.htm]

This space is provided for your personal and/or support group notes.
PLEASE immediately record your ideas, insights, and inspirations as they occur to you.

The Psychoneuroimmunology Research Society (PNIRS) is a leading international organization for researchers in the fields of psychology, neurosciences, immunology, pharmacology, psychiatry, behavioral medicine, and infectious diseases who are interested in the relationship between behavior and health. The Society's website is www.pnirs.org and its official journal is "Brain, Behavior and Immunity."

Other academics in this field are discussed in this Report.

As important as these scholarly foundations are for the scientific credibility of the field, Psychoneuroimmunology is far more than just an academic subject. Mind-body science has such vital broad-based practical uses that the general public has enthusiastically embraced it as well. Checking how cancer book sales rank on Amazon.com reveals the growing popularity of titles about this subject (including some of the books mentioned in this Report).

This extended discussion of PNI is important in order to understand fundamental premises underlying the *Cancer Report*. All of the contributors rely on one or more aspects of the science of Psychoneuroimmunology. Their work reveals the ASTONISHING POSSIBILITIES OF MIND-BODY TREATMENTS.

Who Can Benefit and How

We hope that the format of this Report (including the special workbook pages) will be useful for patients, healthcare professionals, support group facilitators, and other support persons. We encourage the development and will assist with the formation of support/study groups led by licensed, qualified healthcare professionals. The *Cancer Report* is a beginning, not an end. It is the beginning of your permanent recovery from cancer and its goal is to increase the recovery rate in each community while at the same time reducing the number of new or recurring cancer cases reported. We can help with establishing each community's short and long range goals and with the action plan to accomplish them.

This space is provided for your personal and/or support group notes.
PLEASE immediately record your ideas, insights, and inspirations as they occur to you.

The website for the *Cancer Report* is: www.cancer-report.com. This site will provide useful material about starting or joining a support/study group in your area.

On the last page of this Report you will find an order form should you wish to order additional copies.

We hope all those who read these detailed studies will learn that non-invasive methods of treatment can work for them as it has for the thousands of individuals whose success stories are the basis of the research in this Report. The proof presented is your roadmap to wellness. We encourage you to use this Report as a potentially powerful healing tool for conquering your cancer and achieving a full and permanent recovery.

Surviving cancer is also a beginning, not an end. All who have experienced the ravages of cancer and have used this science of mind-body therapy successfully know that their story is not finished. Mastering your cancer is only the first step in understanding how your experience can be of enormous service to others beginning to travel this same path. We hope you will embrace this opportunity to serve and share what you have learned.

This space is provided for your personal and/or support group notes.
PLEASE immediately record your ideas, insights, and inspirations as they occur to you.

Part I

Scientific Research
&
Case Studies

This space is provided for your personal and/or support group notes.
PLEASE immediately record your ideas, insights, and inspirations as they occur to you.

1

CHAPTER 1

Why You Should Read
CANCER REPORT

Stop right now and give thanks for how this Report found its way into your hands... because according to these medical doctors, psychologists, cancer foundations, and healing centers, you are now holding research and clinical evidence that will reveal to you the true causes and cures of most cancers.

The purpose of the *Cancer Report* is to provide the latest information, tools, and resources needed by all those who have cancer, fear cancer or worry that it will return.

We hear some of you saying, "I do not fall into any one of those three categories"... and we say to you, 1) please pass this on to someone who does; 2) please consider the following alarming statistics... just in case you are not aware.

1 in 3 females will have cancer during her lifetime.
1 in 2.5 men will have cancer during his lifetime.

These are your chances of getting cancer and...

If you follow only conventional procedures, the odds are that you will die of cancer. And if you exclusively rely on modern cancer treatments, you will suffer invasive, painful, nauseating, expensive modern medical treatments (with some loss of income, too) while at the same time developing more emotional issues as a direct consequence of all these procedures.

These are the generally expected results for controlling cancer if you use only traditional treatments and screenings... and choose to ignore the amazing successful research presented and documented in the *Cancer Report*... based on 70,000 cancer cases over the last thirty years.

This space is provided for your personal and/or support group notes.
PLEASE immediately record your ideas, insights and inspirations as they occur to you.

1

The good news is that thousands of people are proving that they can have a complete and permanent recovery from cancer—sometimes even if it is in the final stage.

It is quite profound and irrefutable when you fully realize that all of these MD's and counselors who have contributed to this Report have come to the same basic astounding conclusions regarding cancer… separately….

And here it all is, summarized for you and your loved ones.

Here is Hope.
Here are the Facts.
Here are your Choices.

All you need to do is read this Report and take action by using the "Patients Personal Recovery Guide" provided in chapter 13.

And then please, please pass it on and encourage others!

With Love, Respect, and Hope,

John R. Voell and Cynthia A. Chatfield

This space is provided for your personal and/or support group notes.
PLEASE immediately record your ideas, insights and inspirations as they occur to you.

2

CHAPTER 2

A Modern Integrative Cancer Practice:
W. Douglas Brodie, MD

2

Why Dr. Brodie?

There are probably hundreds of physicians who now specialize in alternative and integrative treatments for cancer patients, in settings from a small solo office to elaborate and expensive state-of-the-art clinics with residential facilities. Dr. Brodie was chosen for this Report for several reasons. The most important, by far, was his rare and profound understanding (gleaned from a half century of experience) of the importance of addressing the mental/emotional causes that almost always underlie the development of most cancers.

Over the course of fifty years of treating many thousands of cancer patients, Dr. Brodie observed that there were certain personality traits and stressors that were consistently present in these patients. Much of his website is devoted to offering an extraordinarily insightful look at what he has found to constitute "the cancer personality." He also includes a list of what he has come to believe are the seven most important "success factors" in determining whether there will be a positive outcome for a particular patient, again based on decades of observations. With Dr. Brodie's permission, all of this crucial information will be included later in this chapter, exactly as he has written it. This material is something every cancer patient will want to seriously consider.

Although to act upon these concepts requires us to overcome the desire to avoid painful self-examination and catharsis, it also offers real hope for those with the courage to walk this difficult path. Brodie calls this the willingness "to expose and address deep-seated emotions and to resolve long-standing conflicts": the key to true and lasting healing on several levels.

This space is provided for your personal and/or support group notes.
PLEASE immediately record your ideas, insights, and inspirations as they occur to you.

2

A Pioneer in Alternative Cancer Treatment

One of the original and most highly regarded pioneers in the field of integrative cancer treatment, Dr. Brodie has experience and expertise in conventional as well as complementary and alternative treatments. He began focusing exclusively on alternative and integrative medicine in the early seventies, long before the public knew much about this orientation. As his practice began to shift toward alternative cancer treatments, desperate cancer patients from across the country sought his services.

Early on, Dr. Brodie developed several unique procedures for enhancing the immune system in cancer patients. Although he incorporates chemotherapy and radiation, these more traditional treatments are usually given in much smaller amounts than typical. He has found that his additional alternative methods offer substantial protection against the toxic side effects of chemotherapy and radiation.

Because of his courageous stance on medical freedom and the patient's right to choose a personal treatment plan that includes an integrative or alternative approach, Dr. Brodie was brought before the California medical board, which made three unsuccessful attempts to revoke his medical license. Although he was severely criticized by the medical establishment for his non-conventional treatment methods, Dr. Brodie has never had his license revoked.

In 1980 he made the decision to practice exclusively in Nevada, a state with a high number of alternative and integrative cancer clinics, resulting from a less restrictive and more favorable legal climate.

By 1983 Dr. Brodie was appointed by the governor of Nevada to serve on the newly-formed State Board of Homeopathic Medical Examiners. This was only the second such board ever created in the nation. Dr. Brodie continues to be licensed to practice medical homeopathy as well as conventional medicine. He is a much sought-after speaker and teacher and trains other physicians in his treatment protocols.

This space is provided for your personal and/or support group notes.
PLEASE immediately record your ideas, insights, and inspirations as they occur to you.

2

A Conversation With Dr. Brodie

Dr. Brodie had some fascinating things to say when he was interviewed for this chapter. Commenting about how the Brodie Clinic addresses the mental and emotional aspects of disease, he observed that psychological conflicts, particularly suppressed anger, underlie the development of cancer in most of the cases he has treated. He emphasized, "Suppressed anger seems to be, by far, the most common emotional feature of cancer patients in general." He added that this anger "has usually been suppressed for so long that patients either can't bring it out, or don't even realize that it's there… but it's down there somewhere in just about every case. We try to bring these things out and point out that this is really part of the disease, an important part and one that must be addressed."

Dr. Brodie observed that with help most patients do recognize this aspect of their cancer, although there are a few who resist this realization completely and remain in denial. He observed that many males over sixty found the suggestion of a psychological component to their disease to be unacceptable, and this age group, more than any other, refuses psychological support.

The Brodie Clinic protocol for treating cancer generally includes a three-week residential stay in Nevada, with at least one session per week with the clinic's psychologist, who is very experienced in addressing and resolving these emotional issues. Upon the conclusion of the treatment, every effort is made to find an appropriate therapist to support the patient at home and this is emphasized as essential for long-term healing and preventing relapse.

Dr. Brodie adds, "And with every visit with me, I'm constantly reinforcing what the psychologist is doing with them (the patients), although I try not to overwhelm them." In this way, he functions almost as a therapist as well, because he has found this support to be an essential component of long-term healing, every bit as important as the medical treatments he offers.

Brodie continued, "We provide all the physical interventions possible, but we cannot neglect the psychological. It's a much-neglected aspect of cancer care, even by the best alternative physicians out there, and that needs to change. The emotional aspects of cancer cannot be ignored."

This space is provided for your personal and/or support group notes.
PLEASE immediately record your ideas, insights, and inspirations as they occur to you.

2

Physical interventions include various I.V. infusions, IPT or Insulin Potentiation Therapy, and other methods to support and enhance the functioning of the immune system.

He emphasized, however, that even with tumor destruction, "The immune system must still be regenerated and the emotional issues addressed, or the cancer will likely recur at some point."

A member of Dr. Brodie's staff also offered an observation, in a recent conversation, on the profound effect of stress on the immune system caused by unresolved negative relationships. One cancer patient at the clinic was being closely monitored and her immune system measured at 70% activity. On Monday following a difficult weekend visit from a family member, this number had dropped to 10%. All of this was scientifically documented at the clinic. How many cancer patients have watched their immune systems falter and never made this type of connection?

Articles and Lectures by Dr. Brodie

"The Cancer Personality: Its Importance in Healing"

Evidence of a relationship between cancer and personality type has existed for centuries. In dealing with many thousands of cancer patients over the past twenty-eight years, it has been my observation that there are certain personality traits that are rather consistently present in the cancer-susceptible individual. These characteristics are as follows:

1) Being highly conscientious, dutiful, responsible, caring, hard working, and usually of above average intelligence.

2) Exhibiting a strong tendency toward carrying other people's burdens and toward taking on extra obligations, often "worrying for others."

3) Having a deep-seated need to make others happy, tending to be "people pleasers." Having a great need for approval.

4) Often having a history of lack of closeness with one or both parents, sometimes later in life, resulting in lack of closeness with spouse or others who would normally be close.

This space is provided for your personal and/or support group notes.
PLEASE immediately record your ideas, insights, and inspirations as they occur to you.

2

5) Harboring long-suppressed toxic emotions, such as anger, resentment and/or hostility. Typically the cancer-susceptible individual internalizes such emotions and has great difficulty expressing them.

6) Reacting adversely to stress, often becoming unable to cope adequately with such stress. Usually experiencing an especially damaging event about two years before the onset of detectable cancer. The patient is unable to cope with this traumatic event or series of events, which comes as a "last straw" on top of years of suppressed reactions to stress.

7) Showing an inability to resolve deep-seated emotional problems and conflicts, usually arising in childhood; often even being unaware of their presence.

Typical of the cancer-susceptible personality, as noted above, is the long-standing tendency to suppress "toxic emotions," particularly anger.

Usually starting in childhood, this individual has held in his/her hostility and other unacceptable emotions. More often than not, this feature of the affected personality has its origins in feelings of rejection by one or both parents. Whether these feelings of rejection are justified or not, it is the perception of rejection that matters, and this results in a lack of closeness with the "rejecting" parent or parents, followed later in life by a similar lack of closeness with spouses and others with whom close relationships would normally develop. Those at higher risk for cancer tend to develop feelings of loneliness as a result of their having been deprived of affection and acceptance earlier in life, even if this is merely their own perception. These people have a tremendous need for approval and acceptance, developing a very high sensitivity to the needs of others while suppressing their own emotional needs.

These good folks become the "caretakers" of the world, showing great compassion and caring for others, and going out of their way to look after the needs of others. They are very reluctant to accept help from others, fearing that it may jeopardize their role as caretakers or that they might appear to have too much self-concern. Throughout their childhood they have typically been taught "not to be selfish," and they take this to heart as a major lifetime objective. All of this benevolence is highly commendable, of course, in our culture, but must be somehow modified in the case of the cancer patient. A distinction needs to be

This space is provided for your personal and/or support group notes.
PLEASE immediately record your ideas, insights, and inspirations as they occur to you.

2

made here between the "care-giving" and the "care-taking" personality. There is nothing wrong with care-giving, of course, but the problem arises when the susceptible individual derives his/her entire worth, value and identity from his/her role as "caretaker." If this shift cannot be made, the patient is stuck in this role, and the susceptibility to cancer greatly increases.

As noted above, a consistent feature of those who are susceptible to cancer appears to be that they "suffer in silence," and bear their burdens without complaint. Burdens of their own as well as the burdens of others weigh heavily, often subconsciously as well as consciously, upon these people because they, through a lifetime of suppression, internalize their problems, cares and conflicts. The care-free extrovert, on the other hand, seems to be far less vulnerable to cancer than the caring introvert described above.

How one reacts to stress appears to be a major factor in the development of cancer. Most cancer patients have experienced a highly stressful event, usually about two years prior to the onset of detectable disease. This traumatic event is often beyond the patient's control, such as the loss of a loved one, loss of a business, job, home, or some other major disaster. The typical cancer victim has lost the ability to cope with these extreme events, because his/her coping mechanism lies in his/her ability to control the environment. When this control is lost, the patient has no other way to cope.

Major stress causes suppression of the immune system, and does so more overwhelmingly in the cancer-susceptible individual than in others. Thus personal tragedies and excessive levels of stress appear to combine with the underlying personality described above to bring on the immune deficiency that allows cancer to thrive. These observations have given rise to the term psychoneuro-immunology.

In my experience, one of the most difficult and most important hurdles to overcome in cancer patients is how to make major changes in their lifestyles. Not only is it necessary to make changes in the physical aspects of their lives such as eating habits, but also major changes need to be made in the way they react to stress.

The way they react to stress is due largely to the way they think about life There can be no lasting changes of behavior without first having a change in

This space is provided for your personal and/or support group notes.
PLEASE immediately record your ideas, insights, and inspirations as they occur to you.

2

thinking and in belief systems. It is often extremely difficult for these patients to make substantial changes in these ingrained patterns of thought. Many find it too difficult or too disagreeable to make such alterations in their settled way of thinking and reacting. Many likewise find it too unpleasant to make changes in the physical aspects of their life-style, even in the face of life-threatening illness.

In my office patients are counseled to address their problems and to make the appropriate adjustments to the best of their ability. A psychologist with extensive experience in dealing with these unique problems is readily available to our patients.

These patients are encouraged to take charge of their own health and to be active participants in their care. They are urged to learn as much as possible about the disease and all of the treatment options, including the various conventional modalities.

"Success Factors in Dealing with Cancer"

A positive attitude is essential to a successful outcome for all cancer patients. It is absolutely essential that the patient reject the prevailing concept that death from cancer is inevitable, and the belief that conventional medicine offers the only hope for survival.

Success Factors: Certain consistent features or attributes distinguish the successful cancer survivors from those who are less successful. The successful cancer patients, by and large, are those who are:

1) Willing and able to reverse a stressful life-style, to reduce heavy obligations, burdens and anxieties, and who learn to say "No" to those who would lay burdens upon them.

2) Aware of the critical importance of spiritual growth and having faith in God or their concept of a Higher Power.

3) Ready and eager to take charge of their own health care, to study in depth the various alternatives, and to make dietary and other changes in their physical life-style.

4) Able to reject the idea that the diagnosis of cancer automatically means death and that conventional treatment offers the only hope.

This space is provided for your personal and/or support group notes.
PLEASE immediately record your ideas, insights, and inspirations as they occur to you.

2

5) *Willing to accept responsibility for the behavioral factors which led to the disease, to submit to self-assessment, and to make the necessary adjustments and corrections to eliminate these factors.*

6) *Prepare to abandon destructive and "toxic" emotions such as fear, anger, resentment, guilt and self-pity, replacing these with such positive emotions as hope, love, forgiveness, gentleness, confidence, and faith.*

7) *Able to overcome inhibitions, particularly learned restraints which may have prevented full sexual gratification, allowing guiltless and total fulfillment.*

2

Conventional medicine has only recently begun to recognize the connection between the mind and the immune system. The mind is an extremely important aspect of a healthy immune system, healing and freedom from disease.

The surviving cancer patient has a healthy skepticism of the conventional approach to cancer, and questions all of the premises of that approach. He/she is eager to study in depth all treatment modalities without prejudice, then to follow the chosen course or courses with dedication, discipline and common sense.

The cancer survivor is most often one who has accepted and welcomed spiritual growth, one who has developed a close relationship with God or a Higher Power.

The successful cancer patient has confidence and faith in his/her course of action. The long-term cancer survivor is usually the one who is willing to expose and address his/her deep-seated emotional problems and to resolve long-standing conflicts.

The foregoing attributes have been those most frequently associated with victory over cancer. In recent years I have come to the conclusion that these attributes or qualities are virtually indispensable to recovery from cancer. It has further been my experience that if the problems and conflicts discussed at the beginning of this section are not addressed and corrected, the cancer patient will likely not get well.

This space is provided for your personal and/or support group notes.
PLEASE immediately record your ideas, insights, and inspirations as they occur to you.

2

More often than not, neither conventional nor alternative methods alone penetrate deeply enough into the patient's inward nature, so much of which is kept beneath the surface and so much of which underlies that patient's disease. Counseling, prayer, meditation, reaching the deeper dwelling place of feeling— all must be brought to bear to resolve the patient's inner conflicts. These underlying issues must be addressed simultaneously with physical treatment, whether it be conventional, alternative or a combination of therapies. Otherwise, none of these physical modalities will be effective. We must recognize loving energy as an essential part of healing.

2

The Cancer Personality:
A Major Factor In Integrative Care

[The following text is an abstract of a lecture Dr. Brodie presented at the Global Holistic Health Summit in Bangalore, India in January 2003. It is a summary of Brodie's thinking on the importance of addressing the repressed emotional imbalances most of us carry throughout our lives.]

These cancer susceptible individuals often carry long-suppressed toxic emotions, such as anger, resentment and hostility, usually arising in childhood, which have been internalized to such an extent that such individuals have extreme difficulty in bringing these unacceptable emotions to the surface. As with many conditions, whatever goes on mentally, emotionally and spiritually in these people can have a profound effect on their physical health. The immune system in particular is continually under the influence of these factors. Conventional medicine has only just begun to recognize the connection between the mind, the emotions and the immune system.

The foregoing information is incorporated into our holistic and integrative program, utilizing the services of an on-site psychologist with extensive experience in helping cancer patients to resolve their particular conflicts. It has been our consistent observation that those patients who are best able to resolve these issues, along with being willing and able to make other life-style changes, are the most successful cancer survivors.

This space is provided for your personal and/or support group notes.
PLEASE immediately record your ideas, insights, and inspirations as they occur to you.

2

Clinic Information

Most logistical information about the Brodie Clinic is available on the website or with a phone call. The Clinic cancer program is offered daily, but is non-residential and patients use accommodations nearby; a list of options is on the website. Two other physicians work with Dr. Brodie. Diseases other than cancer are treated as well. The standard cancer treatment protocol is three weeks and the cost is comparable to or less than similar clinics.

2

In addition to Psychological Counseling and IPT, therapies offered at the Clinic include:

- Nutritional Guidance
- Vitamin-Mineral Infusions
- Biological Response Modifiers
- Immune System Evaluation
- Immune Enhancement Therapy
- Hypoglycemic Therapy
- Cytokines
- Megadose Ascorbate Infusions
- Chelation Therapy
- Homeopathy
- Oxygenation Therapy
- Ultra Violet Blood Irradiation
- Darkfield Microscopy

Contact Information

The Brodie Clinic
6110 Plumas Suite B, Reno, NV 89509
Phone: 775-829-1009
Fax: 775-829-9330
Website: www.drbrodie.com

This space is provided for your personal and/or support group notes.
PLEASE immediately record your ideas, insights, and inspirations as they occur to you.

3

CHAPTER 3

The Success of Mind-Body Therapy:
Susan Silberstein, PhD

"It is more important to know what kind of patient has the disease than to know what kind of disease the patient has."
—Sir William Osler, the Father of Modern Medicine

3

How Personal Tragedy Led to a Lifetime's Work:
25,000+ Clients

Dr. Susan Silberstein founded The Center for Advancement in Cancer Education in 1977, following her young husband's death at age 31 from a rare form of spinal cord cancer. She did so out of her burning desire to make a difference so others would not have to experience the pain, confusion, and frustration she went through in trying to find options for him: "Not because I had any score to settle with the cancer establishment or with his doctors, who were all terribly sincere… it was because I was already intellectually persuaded there had to be other approaches." She continues to serve as the Center's Executive Director. Susan is also a member of the Education Advisory Committee at The National Foundation for Alternative Medicine in Washington, DC.

Susan has counseled more than 25,000 cancer patients at the Center without ever charging a fee [the Center is a 501(C)(3) non-profit organization operating on a donation basis]. She also lectures extensively around the country on cancer prevention as well as alternative and complementary therapies. Susan teaches and serves as a consultant for medical and nursing schools and has participated in numerous national and international symposia. She has created and coordinated hundreds of conferences on mind-body, immunological, and nutritional topics for oncology patients, as well as twenty conferences and numerous "in service" sessions on these topics for health professionals. Susan is the

This space is provided for your personal and/or support group notes.
PLEASE immediately record your ideas, insights, and inspirations as they occur to you.

3

Editor of "Immune Perspectives" magazine and the creator and narrator of the excellent video "Breast Cancer: The Diet Connection." She has just written *Hungry For Health*, a recipe/nutrition book comprising the four basic principles of healthful eating for optimal health, disease prevention, and disease reversal.

During the course of her counseling work with thousands of cancer patients, Susan has learned much. She told us, "I may not know everything about cancer treatments, but I do know cancer patients!" Indeed, she probably knows cancer patients better than anyone else doing this work! In a one-on-one setting, Susan and her volunteer staff help clients recognize life issues and other impediments to healing. The Center also offers individualized recommendations for treatments, facilities, physicians and/or other practitioners. She continues to personally handle the most challenging cases.

During an interview for the book *Remarkable Recovery: What Extraordinary Healings Tell Us About Getting Well and Staying Well* (by Caryle Hirshberg), Susan described the process she employs with clients. She looks carefully at each patient's physical, financial, and geographic limitations. She and her volunteers analyze physiological status and nutritional habits, attitudes and beliefs, mental and emotional status, goals and social support systems.

> *We look at their mental or emotional readiness for a certain treatment approach. We never tell patients what they should or shouldn't do. We ask them what their doctors have told them, what the doctors are offering them, how they feel about the doctor, what they feel comfortable doing in the conventional or unconventional medical world. Then we start offering them resources. You can't believe how intimately involved I can get with a patient at the end of an hour. I know stuff about them that they swore they never told anybody. It's not because I'm a brilliant psychologist. I think it's because I've learned so much from what the other thousands of patients have taught me.*

The Importance of Mind-Body Medicine/Psychoneuroimmunology

Susan described the available science and research on the mind-body aspects of cancer and the field of Psychoneuroimmunology (PNI) as voluminous. She explains to patients that PNI refers to the field of science relating to how

This space is provided for your personal and/or support group notes.
PLEASE immediately record your ideas, insights, and inspirations as they occur to you.

3

thoughts and emotions directly affect the immune system. When clients are open to hearing about this topic, Susan generally recommends they start by reading *Cancer as a Turning Point* by psychotherapist Lawrence LeShan, PhD, who has worked with cancer patients for fifty years. Over the past thirty years, approximately half of Dr. LeShan's cancer patients with a poor prognosis have gone into remission… and are still alive—an amazing statistic! [Note: More of Dr. LeShan's work is discussed in chapter 5 of this Report.]

Susan can quote references from numerous books, studies, and authors:

> *PNI is a field that is over a quarter of a century old—it's been around as long as I've been involved in this field. There is research now from everywhere in the world about the emotional patterns that influence the etiology [cause of disease] and the outcome of cancer. I could literally spend the next several hours just telling you the names of researchers and some of the things they've done. I don't even know where to start. This is huge!*

She likes to discuss the topic of spontaneous remission because it gets clients excited about the possibilities for them. It helps if they know that there are literally thousands of cancer patients who have fully recovered primarily because of an emotional change. Caryle Hirshberg's book *Spontaneous Remission: An Annotated Bibliography* contains 1,574 cases. A 1966 book by Everson and Cole on spontaneous remission contained information about 1,900 validated cases through 1960 alone.

Susan described some quick scenarios she recalled from these works, such as a uterine cancer patient with two weeks to live who hated her husband but felt helpless to leave her marriage. He suddenly died and she got well. There was also a testicular cancer patient who had sexuality problems relating to his mother. As soon as he worked through these issues enough to get married, his cancer disappeared.

How does Susan broach this very delicate subject of emotional causes that may contribute to the development of a client's cancer? Very carefully.

> *I try never to pin something on people. Finger pointing can be very disturbing for people and there's a lot of that out there. There are a "host" of factors that can cause cancer. Cancer is usually the result of a combination of factors: the mental/emotional, the genetic, the physical, and the*

55

This space is provided for your personal and/or support group notes.
PLEASE immediately record your ideas, insights, and inspirations as they occur to you.

3

environmental. When you get several aspects together, that's potentially deadly.

Susan further explained how she brings up the mental and emotional aspects when she sees that they likely apply with a client:

For example, when I see a strong correlation with a probable emotional pattern I will say, "You know, a large number of my _____(fill in the type of cancer) clients seem to have similar types of stress in their lives. I wonder if this is an area you would like to look at? Is there anything in your situation that you would interpret as stressful?" If they give me the go ahead, I'll go as deep as they will follow. Once I get my foot in the door, I let experience tell me how hard I can push.

She added that she has been a contributing factor to the termination of quite a few destructive relationships, the moving of clients to entirely new and supportive living situations and locations, even complete changes of careers—and many other life-affirming choices positively influencing the course of their diseases.

In describing her counseling role with clients, Susan focuses on "elucidating the areas that are fertile for change, seeing which they choose to address, and then coaching them to find the most economical ways to do so. Economical in terms of their financial, logistical, and geographical limitations." She often only gets one or two hours with a client, but by listening closely, inevitably it only takes a short time to find out who they are, how they think, and to encourage them to begin to open up. Those who are most willing to talk about their personal issues, about what is missing in their lives, about why they think they got sick, will most likely do best in overcoming their illness. Susan stated, "They all come in with an agenda… which therapy is the best to treat my cancer? I say—We have many therapies, who are you? Then we can begin to find the answers together."

When she first began counseling patients twenty-eight years ago, Susan thought that poor diet and nutritional factors were the most likely cause of cancer, and that changing these patterns was the most important action a patient could take. While diet is still extremely relevant, she has now come around nearly 180 degrees in her thinking. If possible, she will take patients down a

This space is provided for your personal and/or support group notes.
PLEASE immediately record your ideas, insights, and inspirations as they occur to you.

3

path that analyzes what is going on in their heads first. She noted that she finds it is much more important to talk to patients about what is "eating" them, rather than what they are actually eating. "If patients are willing to address both issues, then they have a strong formula for success," she noted.

Susan related the story of one of the first patients she met who showed her where her theories might need to shift. A man who had had spinal cancer came to her and related a medical prognosis that would leave him a quadriplegic within six months. He decided to go on a cruise, where he met a "guru" who told him to begin meditating and that "the cancer began in your mind so that's where you'll have to go to get rid of it." He began to practice meditation several times a day. When he returned home, he did some intense psychological work, got a divorce, quit his job, and his cancer went into remission. Susan remembers being confused with this, since she knew he had not changed his diet at all. It was an "aha" experience for her as well.

Who Gets Cancer—and Why

Dealing with the mental and emotional factors surrounding the development of cancer is not just about studying coping styles and stress management techniques. It goes to the very essence of who these patients are. Susan states, "Why people get cancer is the most fascinating and pregnant field for the prevention of cancer that we have today."

Susan has written about the *Psychological Aspects of Persons with Malignant Process* with John W. Rhinehart, MD. As with other contributors to this Report, she has noticed a common pattern of traumatic loss within the six to eighteen month interval immediately prior to the cancer's manifestation. You will also notice many similarities with Dr. Douglas Brodie's characteristics of the "cancer personality" covered in chapter 2 of this Report.

> *Researchers are beginning to recognize that emotional stress plays an enormous role in susceptibility to malignancy. The following characteristics of the "cancering person" are often manifest throughout lifelong patterns— with the exception of the first item. These constitute what might be called "the cancer personality."*

This space is provided for your personal and/or support group notes.
PLEASE immediately record your ideas, insights, and inspirations as they occur to you.

3

Susan's observations about these characteristics are summarized below:

1) *Despair after significant loss. This can be the loss of a person, a job or possession that was central to life—6 to18 months before diagnosis.*

2) *Selflessness. A limited awareness of one's own needs and desires. This has also been described by Charles Renninger as PNS (Pathological Niceness Syndrome). It involves continual catering to another's needs or expectations, guilt associated with fulfilling one's own needs, and lack of acceptance of self. These people are harmonizers, attempting to keep the peace at all costs.*

3) *Suppression of negative emotions such as anger, resentment, rage, hostility, etc. There is a sense of inappropriateness with the expression of these feelings in any manner.*

4) *Inability to form deep emotional relationships or a preponderance of negative, toxic relationships, especially with family.*

5) *A sense of an inability to change the conditions of one's life. Feeling there are no options, a lack of control, hopelessness of the situation. Also a sense of victimization and passiveness. This leads to frustration and ultimately to depression.*

6) *A conscious or unconscious feeling that one does not deserve happiness or success—or even life itself.*

7) *A conscious or unconscious desire to gain, through the legitimate avenue of serious illness, the attention that one could not receive for other reasons. There could be a vested interest in maintaining the disease for manipulative reasons.*

When questioned about whether she had observed similar patterns between certain types of emotional stress and where cancer manifested, Susan said, "After talking to hundreds if not thousands of patients with a particular form of cancer, I've informally observed this—yes—**I've seen some powerful connections between emotional patterns and where the cancer showed up especially when these emotional patterns have been intensified over the last few years.**"

This space is provided for your personal and/or support group notes.
PLEASE immediately record your ideas, insights, and inspirations as they occur to you.

3

Susan's comments and some corresponding cases are summarized below; they provide ideas you may want to consider for your type of cancer. Her astute and thought-provoking observations could constitute a book in itself. **Remember, these correlations are much more complex than the short descriptions we are able to include in this Report. There are generally many synergistic factors that influence the development or remission of cancer. It is not necessarily true that persons with the following emotional patterns will develop cancer or fail to recover from it.**

Lymphoma: Almost all lymphoma patients live in some type of extremely stressful situation. This is usually job-related and they hate their work, or it could be that they hate the environment in which they are living. For example, a person may live in an apartment in a large city, while longing for the country. Many prison inmates develop lymphoma.

Breast Cancer: Susan noted that she has counseled over ten-thousand breast cancer patients. In 99% of the cases, she observed a pattern of lack of nurturing, many times involving a male. Sometimes the problem is inadequate self-nurturing, often present since childhood, and repeated later in life in a relationship. The woman's perception is emotional distancing from the person from whom she is expecting or needing nurturing.

Prostate Cancer: This cancer is similar to breast cancer and usually represents a lifelong pattern of lack of nurturing, often involving females. The result is reflected in the man's incapacity to experience emotional intimacy (both giving and receiving). His perception is emotional distancing from the person from whom he is expecting or needing nurturing. In many cases, suppressed anger, resentment, and/or worry about a partner's unwillingness to be intimate or his inability to perform is present.

Colon and Liver Cancer: This type of cancer relates, along with liver cancer, to repressed anger and resentment (usually since childhood, but generally spanning many years). It may also reflect an inability to let go of these issues.

Kidney Cancer: This cancer involves a situation of very deep patterns of worry, anxiety, and fear, especially fear of failure, and child-like feelings of shame in the face of criticism.

This space is provided for your personal and/or support group notes.
PLEASE immediately record your ideas, insights, and inspirations as they occur to you.

3

Cervical/Uterine Cancer: These forms of cancer can relate to a woman's negative feelings about her sexual experiences and/or behaviors. The predominant emotion is often guilt concerning rape, child molestation, prostitution, unwanted pregnancies, and/or abortions, etc.

Throat Cancer: This kind of cancer usually relates to stifled self-expression and inability to speak up for oneself.

Ovarian Cancer: The ovaries are the most creative organs of the woman's body. This is generally about major creativity that is suppressed or repressed throughout life. It can also be about mothering issues; these women often had disapproving or absent mothers, or they perceive themselves as failures at mothering.

Lung Cancer: This cancer is related to self-expression issues and is an outlet for all kinds of repressed emotions. It often involves frustration over the inability to control others' and/or one's own circumstances, and suppression/repression of self expression relating to this lack of control.

Multiple Myeloma: This is cancer of the bone marrow, which is the deepest place one can go in the body. The Hebrew word for "bone" is the same as the word for "self." Susan has never seen an exception: this cancer is related to issues of very deep, unexpressed, unresolved grief that goes to the very essence of who people are and how they define themselves. It may be related to a situation that the patient has spent a lot of time grieving about in some way.

Susan also shared stories about long-term exceptional cancer survivors who turned their cancers completely around by making some very basic changes in their stress levels, emotional states, and life situations:

Marian was diagnosed in 1985 as a breast cancer patient. She was a victim of incest and had been abandoned by her entire family of alcoholics. She joined a 12-step program, completed the highly acclaimed *A Course In Miracles* (designed and "scribed" by Dr. Helen Schucman), and did "a lot of personal work." She fully recovered.

Gary was diagnosed in 1995 with aggressive metastatic prostate cancer. He had a violent and abusive wife. After a lot of counseling and after ending his marriage, he fully recovered. Of note is the fact that Gary refused all conventional treatment.

This space is provided for your personal and/or support group notes.
PLEASE immediately record your ideas, insights, and inspirations as they occur to you.

3

Jennifer was diagnosed with inoperable kidney cancer in 1985 and given three months to live. She was made to feel inadequate and unworthy her entire life by her parents. She immersed herself in "heavy psychotherapy" and fully recovered.

David was diagnosed in 1985 with metastatic colon cancer. He had long suppressed anger first towards his father and later towards his wife. He did personal therapy, studied *A Course In Miracles,* and fully recovered.

Sam was diagnosed in 1993 with malignant melanoma that metasta-sized to his lungs. He had carried strong resentment towards his parents his entire life. They had tried to force him into the family business while he wanted to be a musician. Sam did psychotherapy, quit his job, went into the music field, and fully recovered.

George, a medical doctor, contracted colon cancer that metastasized to his lungs. He was a hospital president who was extremely angry, even furious about the challenges presented by the healthcare industry, and hated being forced to interface among the industry, the staff, his board, and the hospital administration. When Susan asked George, "Where are you and what are you doing when you feel totally alive?," he described a forty-acre property with gardens he owned in Oregon. He only visited once a year or so, but loved it. Although this was a highly unusual situation (only five minutes into their very first conversation), Susan felt comfort-able enough to suggest that George consider quitting his job and moving to Oregon. He went! He fully recovered and is living a very different and happier life.

Ellen was diagnosed in 1987 with breast cancer. She had a very control-ling abusive husband. When Susan asked her, "What would it take for you to walk away?," Ellen responded, "I think about it all the time, but I can't do anything about it. I have no job, nowhere to go, and I need his insurance." Susan observed that this type of situation is usually the kiss of death for cancer patients. Ellen said, "When I get better, I'll leave." And Susan responded, "No, you don't get it. That's how you get well!" Ellen eventually left her marriage and stayed with friends for a while. She bartered at a co-op (eventually worked there) and slowly built a new life. She upgraded from living in a trailer to an apartment and then bought a house. She fully recovered.

3

This space is provided for your personal and/or support group notes.
PLEASE immediately record your ideas, insights, and inspirations as they occur to you.

3

Susan observed that for many cancer survivors, the only change in their lives has been a dramatic emotional breakthrough. She has seen many cases of these spontaneous remissions over her twenty-eight years of this work, but also many "hard work miracles."

Who Survives Cancer—and Why

Susan has observed certain personality traits common to the overwhelming majority of exceptional cancer survivors. Those patients who are willing to be open and dialogue about their issues allow support people to be of the most help. "And those patients who manage to achieve a balance between cognition, emotions, and behavior are the most likely to outlive their prognosis with quality longevity." She has outlined the following traits common to survivors:

1) *They accept the diagnosis and reject the prognosis: This type of positive attitude implies self-affirmation, being the most authentic person they can be, getting in touch with what is right about them.*

2) *Participation/Initiative/Commitment: This may involve disagreeing with doctors or loved ones and choosing intuitively which treatment feels right according to their own understandings and beliefs. Susan related the story of a patient who needed to make a decision about which treatment to choose. She did not want chemotherapy but was being pressured about it. She told Susan about a dream she had with two pools of water. One was very crowded with women who asked her to join them. That pool looked murky. The other pool was empty but looked pristine, clean, sparkling. The patient decided to dive into the clean pool and it felt wonderful. She chose an alternative treatment, rejected chemotherapy, and recovered.*

3) *Introspection: They use their illness for personal learning and growth, resolving losses, completing grief work, and self-actualizing potential.*

4) *Transformation of personal relationships: This includes learning to receive, making oneself a priority, reconciling conflicts, and purging toxic relationships.*

This space is provided for your personal and/or support group notes.
PLEASE immediately record your ideas, insights, and inspirations as they occur to you.

3

5) *Lifestyle changes: Developing new supportive patterns of diet, exercise, job, and/or living arrangements. Learning to play more and have more fun. Susan often assigns homework that asks clients to begin making a "Fun List." They are to add anything to the list that feels like it would be fun to them and family members are to help. These choices can be outrageous, illogical or impossible, as well as small and seemingly insignificant. Then every night the client chooses one item to do the following day. Susan called this a "fabulous exercise for waking up the healing potential of the body." She continued, "You see, the immune system doesn't know the difference—whether you're actually taking the action, planning it or just thinking about doing it."*

6) *Expression of emotions: Patients need to relate to and deal with both positive and negative emotions that have been suppressed, especially anger and resentment. Susan has clients try to reconnect with the joy of childhood. Just as one can auto-intoxicate if physical detoxification occurs too quickly, so can emotional detox be dangerous if not carefully modulated. Susan suggests that, "If one gets into heavy traumatic emotions, this needs to be handled in a rhythmic, balanced manner using gradual coping techniques." Of course, this implies being under the professional care of a trained clinician. Susan described a three-phase process: recognize the suppressed emotions, remove them from storage, and then get what has been stirred up out of the body. This process can take many forms, including personal therapy, couples counseling, support groups, pastoral counseling, stress management, bodywork, and energy work.*

7) *Life Purpose: Understanding one's place in the spiritual universe. Susan described finding "the one thing that engages them in life, a feeling of purpose, self worth, and meaning, something that is all their own and unique about them—something that they should be completely selfish about." She noted that there are patients who do not want to die, but are not really ready to continue living either. She tries to find ways to engage them in life—to motivate the life force within them.*

If patients really do not want to be here anymore, Susan attempts to clarify that with them as well. Sometimes they are ready to leave and just need a way to get out of their bodies. "Some patients just want to let go and be with a loved one who has passed… we help them to die spiritually at

This space is provided for your personal and/or support group notes.
PLEASE immediately record your ideas, insights, and inspirations as they occur to you.

3

peace because they have gotten in touch with where their spirit really is. Because sometimes it has already crossed over long before the body goes—and that's ok."

Responsibility vs. Response Ability

Susan described the very delicate balance she constantly seeks while showing clients they may have contributed to the development of their cancer, without creating guilt and additional stress for them. This is illustrated by two ways to spell and describe the word "responsibility":

> *There is the traditional way. If you tell patients they have a "responsibility" for creating their illness and their wellness, it implies some blame and leads to guilt. If you spell it the second way—"Response Ability"—you create an awareness that leads to power. This second way can lead to opportunities for the awareness of the many theories, research results, clinical observations relating to emotions and behaviors that might control or reverse their illness…. This process is patient-driven, there is nothing by protocol. We try to present a smorgasbord of options and give clients permission to choose. It is never about guilt and blame; it is always about empowerment! Some clients are ready to embrace certain aspects immediately and some later. It's up to them.*

Susan finished her interview with a story about a cancer patient and her partner who had driven to Philadelphia from New England for a consultation. She quickly surmised there were problems in the relationship as they could not agree on anything and the tension in the air was thick. Susan asked if this happened often and they agreed it was a regular pattern with them.

Susan indicated she was quite concerned for both of them. This was certainly an immediate problem for the cancer patient. Susan explained that based on extensive PNI clinical research on the direct relationship between chronic stress and depressed immune function, it really would not matter which treatment was chosen given this much stress. The conflict would prevent a sufficiently strong immune response. All the stress could not be good for the woman's partner either.

73

This space is provided for your personal and/or support group notes.
PLEASE immediately record your ideas, insights, and inspirations as they occur to you.

3

Susan proposed that the couple spend the six-hour trip home considering alternatives to the current relationship that would work better for them, talking about their relationship in terms of what was in both their best interests. Perhaps they should consider a hiatus from the relationship or couples counseling to remove the very stressful environment they were living in. The woman called Susan the very next day and told her, "Thank you, thank you, thank you! We realized we really weren't happy living together. He moved out this morning and I feel free!" She got better.

Pioneering Excellence in Health Care

Dr. Susan Silberstein is considered a pioneer and leader in the field of holistic health, and was honored as such by The National Foundation for Alternative Medicine on November 16, 2002 at its "Celebrating Excellence" award ceremony in Washington, DC. Her closing remarks included the following prayer: "May the Almighty deliver us from the stubbornness of mind that clings to preconceived ideas. And may He grant us the humility and courage to examine without prejudice new sources of information. Amen." Amen!

Susan's philosophy can be summed up in her statement: "Miracles happen beyond the mainstream of medicine!" And she has witnessed and played a part in many of them.

Dr. Silberstein has created numerous materials available from the Center for Advancement in Cancer Education. Purchase online at the website or call the Center (information provided below). Among them:

Hungry for Health

Dr. Silberstein offers practical lessons in healthful eating that are great for people who want to improve their diet, but may not know where to start or how to proceed. Learn about the four fundamental principles for preventing disease, enhancing wellness or facilitating healing. The book contains 157 "no guilt" recipes with lots of tasty tips and "nutri-notes." The research is based on Susan's twenty-eight years of experience with nutrition and cancer patients, although anyone who wants to improve his/her diet will benefit.

This space is provided for your personal and/or support group notes.
PLEASE immediately record your ideas, insights, and inspirations as they occur to you.

3

"Breast Cancer: The Diet Connection"

Narrated by Dr. Silberstein, this 39-minute presentation (VHS or DVD) outlines key dietary steps to help prevent breast cancer, prevent its recurrence, or support patients during and after treatment. Based on published scientific evidence and over twenty-five years of experience with thousands of women, this recording reviews food and beverage choices which contribute to, or protect against, the disease.

"Kitchen Chemotherapy"

Based on thousands of articles published in the scientific literature documenting the relationship between diet and cancer survival, this 79-minute CD highlights a dozen advantages of implementing nutrition in a cancer treatment program, outlines foods that promote or suppress tumor growth, and explains the connection between cancer and biological terrain.

Contact Information

Center for Advancement in Cancer Education
300 E. Lancaster Ave., Suite 100, Wynnewood, PA 19096
Phone: 610-642-4810
Email: caceinfo@comcast.net
Website: www.beatcancer.org

The Center is available for phone or in-person consultations. A donation is requested, but no one is turned away.

This space is provided for your personal and/or support group notes.
PLEASE immediately record your ideas, insights, and inspirations as they occur to you.

4

CHAPTER 4

A Cure for Cancer:
Ryke Geerd Hamer, MD

Dr. Ryke Geerd Hamer's theories, based on extensive research involving tens of thousands of cancer patients and his own personal experience, deserve inclusion in this Report because of the profound implications they have for healing disease in the twenty-first century. The basic premise of "The New Medicine" offers real hope and the possibility of a cure for most types of cancer and other diseases as well.

The New Medicine

"Through the millennia, humanity has more or less consciously known that all diseases ultimately have a psychic origin and it [this concept] *became a 'scientific' asset firmly anchored in the inheritance of universal knowledge; it is only modern medicine that has turned our animated beings into a bag full of chemical formulas....*

"The NEW MEDICINE understands the body as a unified organism, a unity, with the psyche being the integrator of all functions of behavior and all areas of conflict, and the brain being the main computer of all behavioral functions, conflict areas and organs, and the sum of the consequences of all these events."

—R.G. Hamer, MD

How It Began:
Dr. Hamer's Personal Story

In 1978, after Dr. Hamer had spent fifteen years as an internist, oncologist, and professor of medicine in Germany and Italy, his son, Dirk, was shot during a random act of violence. Dr. Hamer was awakened during the night with this

This space is provided for your personal and/or support group notes.
PLEASE immediately record your ideas, insights, and inspirations as they occur to you.

4

traumatic news. He attended his dying son for three months, remaining in a state of shock and disbelief. Within a year of his son's death Dr. Hamer developed testicular cancer. As a scientist who had been healthy his entire life, he began to search for what seemed to be a plausible connection between his illness and the painful shock of his son's unexpected murder. Dr. Hamer's wife developed cancer as well. He asked himself whether it could just be coincidence that all of this had happened. Thus began Dr. Hamer's journey toward the complete rethinking of long-accepted medical theories about how and why disease develops within certain individuals, how healing really happens, and why so often recovery does not occur when patients rely on conventional medical treatments.

The Legacy of a New Medicine

I believe that the knowledge of the New Medicine is the legacy of my dead son, Dirk. Through his death I myself became ill with cancer. With an honest heart, I have the authority of this legacy to pass on to all those stricken with disease so that they, with the help of the New Medicine, can understand their disease, overcome it, and recover their health.

Dr. Hamer continued practicing as the Chief of Internal Medicine at a gynecology/oncology clinic at Munich University in Germany, even as he was fighting his own battle with cancer. He then began to look much more deeply into his patients' stories and test results. In every case, Dr. Hamer found he could trace the development of cancer to a severe emotional shock or loss that generally occurred within a year or two before the diagnosis. He called these triggering events the "Dirk Hamer Syndrome" or DHS events in honor of his son.

I had the opportunity to study female patients with cancer and to compare my findings to see if their mechanism was the same as mine; if they, too, had experienced such a terrible shock. I found that all of them, without exception, had experienced the same type of biological conflict as I had. They were able to recollect the shock, the resulting sleeplessness, weight loss, cold hands, and the beginning of tumor growth.

Furthermore, the shock must be unexpected; if we are prepared in some manner for the shocking event, we will not become ill, Dr. Hamer believes. Even more

This space is provided for your personal and/or support group notes.
PLEASE immediately record your ideas, insights, and inspirations as they occur to you.

4

remarkably, he discovered that every biological conflict leaves a visible shadow in the brain (confirmed in every case without exception by a brain CT scan) in the exact brain relay corresponding to the organ or body structure manifesting the disease. Dr. Hamer discovered that the nature of the conflict predetermines the organic site for disease and that every disease has two distinct components: the "conflict/active phase" and the "healing/resolution phase." These are separated by the exact moment when the biological conflict is resolved. Hamer called this "The Iron Rule of Cancer."

He soon began to correlate his theories with other diseases in addition to cancer. The result of his research is the creation of the "Disease Chart," which accurately describes the biological conflict cause of each disease, the exact focal location in the brain, how the disease manifests in the "conflict/active phase," and how it is revealed in the "healing phase." (This chart is not yet available.) Should Hamer's theories continue to receive scientific corroboration, their development may indeed constitute the foundation for a New Medicine in the world.

What is a Biological Conflict?

"Cancer does not begin in the body; cancer begins in the brain."

According to information contained on The New Medicine website, a "biological conflict" is explained as follows:

A biological conflict is a very primal response to an event in a person's life that completely catches [him] off guard. In fact, most people describe this event as feeling as if they were struck by lightning, they develop cold hands and feet, lose their appetite, can't sleep, their mind keeps dwelling on the trauma, and they have trouble talking to anyone about it. These conflicts, in order to qualify as biological in nature, must be unanticipated and can involve a separation from a loved one, a territorial loss, a self-devaluation, a profound fear, a fight over something that we believe rightfully belongs to us, injuries inflicted through accidents or harsh words, or even a fear for our lives or the life of a loved one. The list goes on. These biological responses are preprogrammed into our brains and are responsible for creating most of the disease states we are familiar with today.

And how do "spontaneous remissions" happen in nature? In exactly the same manner as a longer term healing process. When the patient's biological conflict

This space is provided for your personal and/or support group notes.
PLEASE immediately record your ideas, insights, and inspirations as they occur to you.

4

situation finally gets resolved—whether naturally as life changes and adaptation occurs, or after significant conscious effort—then the turning point is reached. In many cases, this healing process is not without its challenges and dangers as well, but the tide has definitely turned in the right direction.

Years of Frustration and Rejection

This theory, well researched with twenty thousand case studies and validated with CAT scans (computerized axial tomography: an image of the soft tissues of the body), was something completely new within standard medical practice. When Dr. Hamer presented his discoveries to his colleagues, they demanded that he deny his findings or leave the university immediately. He chose the latter course—and continued his research—although the unjust dismissal haunted him for years. And the situation was to get even worse.

Dr. Hamer next submitted his research to the University of Tubingen in Germany in October 1981 as a post-doctoral thesis. His primary intent was to create the opportunity for his results to be tested as soon as possible so they could begin to benefit cancer patients. In May 1982 the university rejected Dr. Hamer's work without testing even a single case for reproduction—and to this date the university continues to refuse testing. In the ensuing years, he repeatedly attempted to open a clinic where patients could utilize his methods, and each time he was legally prevented from doing so.

The criticism (perhaps "persecution" would not be too strong a word) reached its peak in 1986 when an action was begun to stop Dr. Hamer from practicing medicine on the basis that he "failed to deny his findings and failed to convert to the tenets of official medicine." This judgment was handed down after a single hearing. Dr. Hamer was subsequently forbidden to talk to patients and he was advised, at age 51, to find a new profession, unrelated to medicine. He was even jailed for eighteen months, and charged with "practicing medicine without a license" for providing information to patients about his "New Medicine." His career as a physician appeared to be over.

Dr. Hamer continued his research on a limited basis, denied any kind of financial, technical or administrative support. He finally, successfully, took the University of Tubingen to court and the university was ordered to conduct

This space is provided for your personal and/or support group notes.
PLEASE immediately record your ideas, insights, and inspirations as they occur to you.

4

studies about Dr. Hamer's findings. To date, Tubingen has not done so. Since he believes very strongly that current methods for treating cancer (surgery, chemotherapy, and radiation) are barbaric and completely ineffective on any kind of long-term basis, he has very few supporters within the conventional medical community.

An Amazing 31,000 Patients Studied by 1997

As incredible as it sounds, Dr. Hamer and his supporters describe their series of empirical findings (based on 31,000 case studies) as ALL (not one exception to the theory has been uncovered) exhibiting this same pattern of disease development. In fact, various supportive studies have now been conducted in several European institutions, the latest being the 1998 examination at the University of Trnava, Slovakia.

[Note: There is a great deal of information of a highly technical nature available about Dr. Hamer's theories and set of five "biological laws," which is not included within this Report. Many of his ideas are diametrically opposed to conventional medical knowledge, such as his statement that tumors cannot metastasize, so be forewarned. You will need to proceed with an open mind.]

Some Powerful Insights Into Breast Cancer

For a fascinating discussion specific to breast cancer, go to the New Medicine website: www.newmedicine.ca/breast.php. This is certainly well worth exploring and seriously considering if you, or someone you love, is dealing with breast cancer. Dr. Hamer proposes that there are two types: breast gland and milk duct (or intra-ductal) cancer. He has found that all breast cancer results from separation conflict of some type and that where it manifests will also depend on whether the woman is right or left-handed. This concept can be summarized as follows:

We do not develop either intra-ductal or breast gland cancer without reason. The specific nature or feeling behind the conflict will determine precisely what brain location will receive the impact of the conflict-shock and whether it will be the duct or the gland affected.

This space is provided for your personal and/or support group notes.
PLEASE immediately record your ideas, insights, and inspirations as they occur to you.

4

Breast gland cancer has to do with the woman's nest in the sense that she has a "worry, quarrel or argument" going on in her nest. The worry could be over a health concern of a loved one, or even being thrown out of the nest by her mother! The overall issue concerned, however, is really a separation from a loved one.

Milk duct cancer has quite specifically to do with the conflict of, "my child, mother, or partner has been torn from my breast." Again it is a separation conflict and the rules of laterality also apply here. To be more precise, a right-handed woman will respond with the left breast if she has a mother-child conflict or a daughter-mother conflict, and will respond with the right breast if she has a partner conflict. Her partners include her life's companion as in husband, a friend, her brother, sister, her father, or even her business partner. The opposite breast will be affected in a left-handed woman.

Something to consider: Dr. Hamer makes the following empowering statement for women suffering from this dreaded cancer, offering the possibility, in resolving any emotional/biological conflicts, to create a healing miracle in their lives:

...The tissue starts to augment from the time of the onset of the actual conflict and will stop growing as soon as the conflict has been resolved.

Hamer's Theories Brought to the United States

As Dr. Hamer's theories are finally being investigated and seriously considered in Europe, so, too, are they beginning to be discussed here in the United States. A new organization, The Meta-Medicine Academy, based in large part on Dr. Hamer's work, was established in California in June 2004 to explore the natural laws that govern disease, health, and healing: the "big picture" around how disease and healing truly happen. This is an education and research organization that will offer seminars and courses, including a certified "health coach" training program for practitioners wishing to specialize in this approach. Meta-Medicine will offer a new model for how our bodies really work. The Academy intends to create no less than "the transformation of medicine and healing towards an integral understanding of the body/mind/spirit environment." This information is from the website www.metamedicine.info and explains the mission further:

The goal of Meta-Medicine is to research and find the causes, processes,

This space is provided for your personal and/or support group notes.
PLEASE immediately record your ideas, insights, and inspirations as they occur to you.

4

relationships, and meaning of disease and health, and to formulate a new foundation of a truly integral health system and medicine. The Meta-Medicine is engaged in answering the deeper questions of health and disease from an integral and more comprehensive point of view.

- *What are the causes of disease?*

- *How exactly does body-mind-spirit work together?*

- *What is the process and flow of a disease?*

- *How do our organisms work as holistic, integral systems?*

- *What biological laws and principles can we research from a meta-level?*

- *What are the phases and cycles of a disease?*

- *What is a healing crisis and when does it appear?*

- *Is there a deeper meaning to all disease?*

- *What therapy works best for what disease in what stage?*

- *How can we define and formulate true holistic health prevention?*

- *How can we use all current healing methods more effectively, with the knowledge of the Meta-Medicine?*

- *What new methods of diagnosis, therapy, and treatment can be developed incorporating the Meta-Medicine?*

There are introductory seminars scheduled in California, Germany, and the United Kingdom. Consult the website for details and to be added to the mailing list if you are interested.

Shadows On The Brain

In conclusion, the following article and summary of Dr. Hamer's work is reprinted with permission from the British newsletter, "What Doctors Don't Tell You," Volume 13, No. 10, January 2003. (www.wddty.co.uk). Pat Thomas, Contributing Editor, is the author of the article.

This space is provided for your personal and/or support group notes.
PLEASE immediately record your ideas, insights, and inspirations as they occur to you.

4

One of the most recent studies on psychosomatic cancer therapy comes from Germany. Over the past ten years, medical doctor, cancer surgeon, and cancer survivor Ryke Geerd Hamer has examined over 20,000 cancer patients with all types of cancer.

Dr. Hamer wondered why cancer never seems to systemically spread directly from one organ to the surrounding tissue. For example, he has never found a cancer of the cervix and cancer of the uterus in the same woman. He also noticed that all his cancer patients seem to have something in common: they had all experienced some kind of psycho-emotional conflict prior to the onset of their disease, a conflict that had never been fully resolved.

On the basis of these 20,000 examinations, Dr. Hamer has come up with some revolutionary information. In all these cases, X-rays taken of the brain by Dr. Hamer have shown a dark shadow somewhere in the brain. These dark spots are located in exactly the same place in the brain for the same type of cancer. There was also a 100 percent correlation between the dark spot in the brain, the location of the cancer in the body, and the specific type of unresolved conflict.

These findings have led Dr. Hamer to suggest that when we are in a stressful conflict that is not resolved, the emotional reflex center in the brain that corresponds to the experienced emotion (for example, anger, frustration or grief) will slowly break down. Each of these emotion centers is connected to a specific organ. When a center breaks down it will start sending the wrong information to the organ it controls, resulting in the formation of deformed cells in the tissue—in other words, cancer cells.

Dr. Hamer also suggests that metastases are not the same as cancer spreading. Metastases are the result of new conflicts that the stress of having cancer, or of having to undergo invasive, painful or nauseating therapies, creates.

When Dr. Hamer started including psychotherapy as an important part of the healing process, he found that when the associated conflict was resolved, the cancer immediately stopped growing at a cellular level. The dark spot in the brain also began to disappear, and the diseased tissue came to be replaced by normal tissue.

This space is provided for your personal and/or support group notes.
PLEASE immediately record your ideas, insights, and inspirations as they occur to you.

4

According to Dr. Hamer, research in Germany, Austria, France, the U.S., and Denmark has confirmed his findings—that emotional conflicts create cancer, and solving the conflicts in question stops the cancer's growth.

Dr. Ryke Geerd Hamer has written several books, including: *Cancer, Disease of the Psyche and Legacy of a New Medicine, Volume 1, The Ontogenetic System of Tumors including Cancer, Leukemia, Psychosis and Epilepsy.*

Interested? Check Out the New Medicine Website
www.newmedicine.ca

If you would like to learn more (and you may need a medical or scientific background to comprehend much of this), a good place to start is the English version of the website (cited above). An English translation of "The Summary of the New Medicine" (Dr. Hamer's 1994 University of Tubingen thesis updated in 2000) can be ordered here. This provides comprehensive documentation of his research. The thesis is described as "dense with material and case studies as well as examples of CT scans of the brain, and the New Medicine interpretation involving the Psyche, Brain, and Organ."

Schedules of lectures and seminars are listed on the website. These are conducted by a New Medicine teacher and therapist trained and approved by Dr. Hamer. The programs are reasonably priced and accessible in the U.S. or Canada.

A Remarkable New Medicine Breakthrough

[Note: This is a nearly literal translation from the original German. Some of the technical data has been omitted and some of the more esoteric translation language has been reworded. You will still get a clear understanding of the writer's style and thoughts, and how the New Medicine made an impressive impact on his life. The original is from www.pilhar.com. Addressed to Dr. Hamer and Helmut Pilhar]

My Way of Learning and Healing From Prostate Cancer

Actually, I was either too old or too young at age 49 to wear diapers in April of 1995. It started with a harmless preventive medical checkup.

This space is provided for your personal and/or support group notes.
PLEASE immediately record your ideas, insights, and inspirations as they occur to you.

4

The PSA-value was too high, so a biopsy was in order—positive. A highly differentiated Adenocarzinom of the prostate was diagnosed. I was very well informed about the treatment and its consequences. "In about two weeks everything will be behind you," and so on. Before everything was over, I wanted to go on vacation and the urologist could understand that. From the urologists, I could find out only a little about the reasons for my illness. They had suspicions, assumptions; also I could not find much in the literature.

Since then I have formed a different opinion.

I processed (like in my job as electro-technician) that if there is a defect, the connections can be traced down to the smallest detail. Never can you lose sight of the overall picture with this type of work. Without a cause the motor does not get hot, without a start the light bulb does not light up, and just to take the light bulb out would mean to operate, use radiation. Then I would loose my job quickly. There must be a reason....

A beam of light appeared. It was an article about the direct connection between the body, brain, and psyche by Dr. Hamer. I was curious and could follow the thinking process....

In the meantime I had talked to Gisela R., who used the help of a non-medical practitioner, and also got a brain-CT of my skull. With my own eyes I could see markings in my brain-CT just like it was described in the book. The radiologist did not point out these markings. I was impressed, such an easy diagnosis, but I just could not grasp it all.

Finally, in January of 1996, I could visit one of Dr. Hamer's seminars.

This is how I found out about the workings, the better diagnosis of the New Medicine in person. My illness was discussed with Dr. Hamer and the other participants. To learn from each other directly is most lively.

In this circle of participants I could talk about my hurt, which I tried to avoid until now. I had, as it is described in much of the literature, guessed a connection between my psyche and body, but something concrete could not have been concluded.

This space is provided for your personal and/or support group notes.
PLEASE immediately record your ideas, insights, and inspirations as they occur to you.

4

It was three years earlier, a sentence my wife spoke, which immediately came to mind in this setting. I had not expected to learn how much this had affected me. I could exactly describe the place it happened.

In a fight, sentences are said which intend to hurt. I am not "free from that" (meaning I do that as well). It was a relief to say this openly and not to be judged morally, it is my subjective experience, and that is what matters.

I now understand stress and regeneration.

Now it was up to me to understand the connections and to live a new way of life. In many talks, with so much new information, I was witness to many successes. The connection could always be confirmed. This way I have also gotten to know people who could not work through their conflicts, which for me is another reason to intensively learn more....

In the brain-CT the previous [marking] has disappeared, left is only a small compression in its place, a scar, which can only be seen with a magnifying glass. I see this as an objective fact, which can be proven. Besides a few months of hormone withdrawal, which I ended when my path was clear, I have not taken any doctor's prescribed medicine.

Nine years have passed: I feel normal, healthy, and well.

I want to specifically thank Dr. Ryke Geerd Hamer for the discovery and the spread of the New Medicine, and his service in the creation.

I also want to thank those, who have "dressed" me on my way. The exchange of experience was and is still helpful today. The experiences, the resistance, and the connections of the New Medicine have dramatically changed my knowledge and impressions about this society. With shock I have experienced the power, which stands in the way of my (our health), and which I only knew from far away lands or from books.

Thank you that www.pilhar.com exists [in German], for information and exchange.

Sincerely,

4

This space is provided for your personal and/or support group notes.
PLEASE immediately record your ideas, insights, and inspirations as they occur to you.

4

Bernd Draeger

P.S. Cancer can be healed—but not fought against.

Contact Information

Website: www.newmedicine.ca

For another website devoted to Dr. Hamer's work (you will have to be tolerant of some unusual English translations), go to:

http://membres.lycos.fr/biologie/english/welcome.htm

4

This space is provided for your personal and/or support group notes.
PLEASE immediately record your ideas, insights, and inspirations as they occur to you.

5

CHAPTER 5

Cancer as a Turning Point:
Lawrence LeShan, PhD

In Chinese, there is no word for crisis; the word that comes closest consists of two symbols: one is for "danger," the other for "opportunity."

"Getting cancer can become the beginning of living. The search for one's own being, the discovery of the life one needs to live, can be one of the strongest weapons against disease."

—Lawrence LeShan

That is a powerful statement you may want to read again!

5

The Father of Mind-Body Therapy

Dr. Lawrence LeShan's therapeutic methods have achieved extraordinary results with advanced cancer patients—irrespective of whatever physical healing choices they have made. Over the past thirty-five years that he has been practicing his unique form of psychotherapy, approximately half of his cancer patients with poor prognoses have experienced long-term remission and many are still alive decades later. Nearly all of these patients dramatically improved their emotional state and quality of life. All cancer patients who want to maximize their odds for survival should at least consider how LeShan's approach might be incorporated into the conventional, complementary or alternative physical healing path he/she has chosen.

Dr. Lawrence LeShan has worked with cancer patients for over fifty years and is referred to as "the father of mind-body therapy" by many in the field. He is a research and clinical psychologist and is the author of more than a dozen books, including three excellent choices for cancer patients: *Cancer as a Turning Point: A Handbook for Cancer Patients, Their Families and Health Professionals; You Can Fight For Your Life: Emotional Factors in the Treatment of Cancer;* and *How to Meditate: A Guide to Self-Discovery.*

This space is provided for your personal and/or support group notes.
PLEASE immediately record your ideas, insights, and inspirations as they occur to you.

5

Cancer as a Turning Point uses patient stories to show how to mobilize the cancer patient's self-healing abilities to augment whatever physical healing program the individual has chosen. The book comes out of a thirty-five year research project involving several thousand people with cancer. It is designed to teach cancer patients and their families, friends, physicians, clergymen, and psychotherapists how to use psychological change to help heal and strengthen the person's compromised immune system.

In the beginning of his career, when he first started working with cancer patients, LeShan utilized the classic psychotherapeutic approach from his training, where the model was to uncover what was wrong with the patient and then determine what could be done. Was there something dark and hidden within the patient's psyche? Could it be brought to light and either cured or compensated for?

LeShan then began to shift his treatment method and his questions. He started asking, "What's right with this person? What ways of being with himself, with others, and with the world will lead him to the greatest enthusiasm and satisfaction in his lives? What would provide a solid reason for being, the kind of meaning and purpose that makes her glad to get out of bed in the morning and glad to go to bed at night—the kind of life that makes her look forward zestfully to each day and to the future?"

With that determined, he and his patient together could begin to move toward embracing that way of being and creating that life. In effect, the definition of psychotherapy has been changed from removing the patient's pain and reducing symptoms to helping patients find their own special "music" that will lead them to the "song" they came to sing in this lifetime. LeShan found that this process could be exhilarating for some and downright terrifying for others, but always beneficial in the end.

He describes the process in the following way:

> Let us suppose we say in effect, to a patient, that your Fairy Godmother will come in that door in a few minutes. She will make you an offer. In six months your inner and outer life can be exactly what you would like it to be so that you would use yourself most completely and have the maximum enjoyment and zest possible. You can change your feelings and your circumstances. There are no limitations on age, sex, education, and so forth. We shall assume that you choose good physical health as a

This space is provided for your personal and/or support group notes.
PLEASE immediately record your ideas, insights, and inspirations as they occur to you.

5

basis and take it from there. There are only two catches. You must tell her in the next five minutes, and this is a once-in-a-lifetime deal. She won't be back after granting your proposal.... You will have just described your heart's deepest desire and where and how you would love to live.

Therapy that is useful for mobilizing cancer patients' immune systems aims at discovering the answer to this question and understanding what has blocked its perception and/or its being lived out as a life-style. And then helping patients move toward it. Very often patients will respond with "I don't know" when asked how they would change their life. The goal then becomes having them accept that this is the most important question at this stage of their life. Mere acceptance of the question and a commitment to finding out the answer frequently have a positive effect on patients' immune systems. I have seen patients who began to respond better and more effectively to their medical protocol when they made and emotionally accepted the commitment.

An individual's special "song" is not expressed, in part, because emotional blockages and pathologies have not been released. These blockages also cause the patient's loss of connection to enthusiasm and joy. Yet when people with cancer have been presented with this concept, LeShan observed that there is generally strong resistance; the objections are usually represented by the following three types of excuses:

> *If I found my own music, it would be so discordant that I wouldn't like it and no one else could stand it either. My own "natural" way of being is ugly and repellent, and I learned a long time ago not to express it if I wanted to have any relationships or be able to live with myself.*

> *If I found my own song and tried to sing it, I would find there was no place in this world for anyone like me. (The major variation here is "I couldn't support myself if I was living the song that is right for me.") And it would be so bitter to know it and not be able to sing it that I'd rather not know.*

> *My own song would have such contradictions built into it that it would be impossible. (As one patient put it, "I'd really like to be a hermit with a harem!")*

This space is provided for your personal and/or support group notes.
PLEASE immediately record your ideas, insights, and inspirations as they occur to you.

5

LeShan continues:

In more than twenty-five years of using this approach, I have seen these reactions many, many times. Yet I have never seen a single person who, finding his or her own song and style, still felt the same. With all the people with whom I have worked, their own song was one that was acceptable to them and others, was possible to play fully in this culture (and to make a living when this was necessary), and increased their human relation-ships and made them more fulfilling. In addition, in every case, the song was socially positive and acceptable. I have never seen an exception to this.

Something Within Us Yearns For Wider Vistas and Broader Skies

5

LeShan coaches patients to take control over their own lives, to search for a life-style that truly suits them and expresses who they are—and then begin to move toward creating that lifestyle. For most, this will entail a complete transformation of how they view themselves, no longer being motivated by what they "should" do, but by what they would enjoy doing. LeShan asks his patients to dig down and ask themselves: "What would truly fulfill me—what style of being, relating, creating would bring me to a life of zest and enthusiasm?" Time and again, he finds that the answer to this question is the very thing that would most profoundly mobilize his patient's immune system against cancer.

Over and over again, I have seen one of two things happen when the total environment of the person with cancer is mobilized for life and his or her inner ecology is thereby changed in a positive way. For some, the patient's life is prolonged, not in an arbitrary way, but in order that there may be more experience of the self, self-recognition, and the recognition—and often fulfillment—of dreams. And then there were the genuine miracles—not magic, but dedicated devotion and hard work which made the cancer a turning point in the person's life rather than a sign of its ending. The more we learn about human biology and psychology, the more we learn about how to change and improve the quality and ambiance of life both internal and external, the more this second result may become common-place. And when it is time to die, we need to understand what our life was about, to know and accept who we have become.

This space is provided for your personal and/or support group notes.
PLEASE immediately record your ideas, insights, and inspirations as they occur to you.

5

A Tale of Two Patients:
How Psychological Change Can Mobilize
A Compromised Immune System

The term "hopeless" should be banished from the cancer patient's vocabulary. There is ALWAYS hope!

Two of LeShan's patient stories illustrate much of what has been related so far. Ethel had metastasized breast cancer and had been told by her doctors that she had approximately two months to live. She sought therapy to deal with her fear in order to maintain her quality of life until the moment of death. It was not difficult to uncover her secret dreams. Ethel yearned to travel, particularly on the ocean, and she had always felt she belonged at sea, jokingly saying that in a previous life, she must have been a sailor.

Her best memories were the ten years she had worked as a saleswoman in an exclusive clothing store, an experience she loved. Even then, Ethel had pored over travel brochures and dreamed of cruises. She became a wife, then a mother, and put away her dreams for what she believed was the reality she was supposed to be living.

Now that Ethel was a cancer patient, she was asked, "Why not travel now?" Her husband was dead, her children grown and independent. She replied that now she was sick and should not leave her excellent medical care. It did not take much convincing to get her to reconsider that rather bleak option. And so Ethel took all her life savings and booked a first class cabin on a long cruise— and off she went, with great excitement and anticipation.

Four months later, she stormed into the doctor's office and shouted, "Here, I've spent all my money. I'm broke—and I'm still alive!" She and the doctor began to laugh, as he pointed out the obvious alternative. He was later able to use connections to get Ethel a job selling in a boutique on an ocean liner, creating a life-style that she absolutely loved. The cancer had shown no signs of increasing and slowly shrank to about half its original size over the years. Ethel had no further medical treatments, but simply went forward, joyfully living a life that she found completely fulfilling and exciting. She sent the doctor a Christmas

This space is provided for your personal and/or support group notes.
PLEASE immediately record your ideas, insights, and inspirations as they occur to you.

5

card every year—no matter where in the world she was.

And then there was Carol, a highly successful executive and a vice-president in a large corporation. Her family was proud of her, her colleagues were envious. The only thing wrong was that Carol hated her life and everything about it. She despised the cutthroat tactics of people who succeeded in her world, disliked the ruthless ambition of her colleagues, and was afraid she might become like them, at some point. In her late thirties, she developed six malignant melanomas on her back and was told her prognosis was extremely poor. Carol left the doctor's office and immediately called LeShan to make an appointment, already committed to do whatever it took to heal.

She soon recognized how her negativity toward her life-style was hurting her. LeShan kept returning the focus from the negative to what Carol liked most in life. Was there any time she had deeply enjoyed her work, had felt at home, fulfilled and happy? When had she felt "the good tired" rather than the "yuck tired" at the end of the day? "When and where had you had those periods in which you suddenly look up, three hours have gone by, you missed lunch and never noticed?" He kept Carol returning to these questions.

Soon she remembered an experience during college when she worked at a center for retraining physically-handicapped adults who had been injured in accidents and were being re-taught living skills. She had been deeply involved in work at the center and loved it. Now Carol considered whether this type of work in special education would fulfill her in the present. But to choose this, she would have to leave her upscale life-style and go back to school—how could she even begin to consider this?

Carol took a couple of evening courses and found that she loved them. To the absolute horror of family and friends, she soon quit her job, sold her penthouse and became a full-time graduate student, eventually becoming the special education teacher and counselor she wanted to be.

After six months of psychotherapy, Carol's melanomas started to shrink. This continued until they completely disappeared and... they have never reappeared. Carol was still cancer-free over twenty years later when LeShan's book *Cancer as a Turning Point* was written.

Carol began to taper off her therapy appointments until finally they stopped altogether. Ten years later, LeShan met her "bounding jauntily down the street."

This space is provided for your personal and/or support group notes.
PLEASE immediately record your ideas, insights, and inspirations as they occur to you.

5

They greeted each other with a big hug, talked for a minute and then both hurried off for appointments. After a couple of steps, Carol turned around and asked, "Do you know why I've stopped staying in touch with you?" He shook his head. She answered, "It's because I've been much too busy living my life to have any time for such nonsense as cancer, psychotherapy, or you!" LeShan's concluding comment really says it all: "For a psychotherapist, this was a combination of the Congressional Medal of Honor and the Nobel Prize. There could not have been a finer reason."

What Actions Can You Take to Shape Your Life So It More Closely Resembles Your Dreams?

Can a cancer patient take on this life-altering work alone, without a therapist or counselor guiding the way? Yes, certainly Greg Anderson was able to do this (see Chapter 11 in this Report). LeShan comments that although patients working alone may not be able to go as deep, nor explore and gain insight to the same degree, yet "great progress can be made, life-styles can be changed greatly and definite positive effects can be made on the immune system." A true commitment to make these changes must be present, even if it forces us to walk through every one of our worst doubts and fears. "Sometimes it can be done alone. Sometimes it takes the help of a psychotherapist."

The final chapter of LeShan's book is a workbook, with twenty-nine exercises designed to help individuals explore who they are and what their ideal life would look like. Most of us do not have any idea where or how to begin this process. These exercises are also great for anyone who wants a more fulfilling life, not just cancer patients who need to stimulate their immune systems. "The immune system is feeble-minded," LeShan says. It follows that if we feel we are unique and worthwhile enough to take care of ourselves, then our immune system will believe us and go to work to do exactly that. If we create extra years of good health and a fulfilling, joyful life living our dreams, then we will have healed not only our bodies, but our hearts and spirits as well.

Cancer as a Turning Point is every bit as relevant and on the cutting edge of our medical knowledge as it was when first published in 1989. We highly recommend it for every cancer patient and for those who work with them in any capacity.

This space is provided for your personal and/or support group notes.
PLEASE immediately record your ideas, insights, and inspirations as they occur to you.

5

Consider with us now, for just a moment, what kind of a world this would be if every one of us had the courage to create these profound changes and embrace a satisfying, joyous life right now… without waiting for a wake-up call like cancer to force us to look at what is so deeply out of balance in our lives. If we all sang our exquisite "songs" together, what kind of perfect harmony would be created around us? What would we "not have any time for" anymore?

[Note: There are two additional sections of the book that should be mentioned. LeShan includes an excellent chapter on meditation and another chapter with great advice about how to find the right therapist.]

Contact Information

Phone: 212-496-9136
Email to Ruth Bolletino: rbolletino@aol.com
Website: www.cancerasaturningpoint.org

Dr. LeShan and his associates offer five-day residential workshops, intensive "marathon" psychotherapy and individual therapy sessions, as well as training in these methods for healthcare professionals. Consult his website or call for details.

This space is provided for your personal and/or support group notes.
PLEASE immediately record your ideas, insights, and inspirations as they occur to you.

6

CHAPTER 6

The Scientific Connection
Between Emotions and Health:
Candace Pert, PhD

"Candace has taken a giant step toward shattering some cherished beliefs held sacred by Western scientists for more than two centuries. Her pioneering research has demonstrated how our internal chemicals, the neuropeptides and their receptors, are the actual biological underpinnings of our awareness, manifesting themselves as our emotions, beliefs, and expectations, and profoundly influencing how we respond to and experience our world."

—Deepak Chopra, MD

(from the Foreword of *Molecules of Emotion: The Science Behind Mind-Body Medicine* by Candace Pert)

The Chicken or the Egg:
The Body or the Mind: Which Comes First?

Dr. Pert's Answer: The "Bodymind"

Dr. Candace Pert rocketed to fame in the scientific world in the early seventies when, as a fledgling neuropharmacologist, she took on the daunting task of finding the opiate receptor for her doctoral dissertation at the Johns Hopkins School of Medicine. For the next decade and a half she headed a laboratory at the National Institutes of Health that published over two hundred scientific articles explaining the discovery of numerous "neuro-peptides." (Peptides and receptors are terms that will be explained later in this chapter.) The groundbreaking work that Pert did with the opiate receptor was later nominated for a Lasker Award, also known as the "American Nobel Prize," awarded annually for outstanding medical research.

This space is provided for your personal and/or support group notes.
PLEASE immediately record your ideas, insights, and inspirations as they occur to you.

6

Pert's discovery of the opiate receptor started a revolution that would later create profound shifts within every field of modern medicine. This discovery would ultimately unite immunology, endocrinology, neuro-physiology, psychology, and biology into a cohesive theory about how our thoughts and emotions are capable of creating wellness or disease in our bodies. This theory would explain and validate what Eastern healing traditions, shamans, energy healers, and most alternative practitioners have understood for eons.

Eastern philosophy states that consciousness precedes reality. Western thought espouses the opposite view and has taught for hundreds of years that consciousness, thoughts, and emotions are products of the physical brain and have little to do with the body or our health. How many times has the statement, "It's all in your head," been given when no logical answer makes sense, thus suggesting that whatever complaint is being reported by the patient is not real. Pert would say it is all in your "bodymind" and it is all-important. She maintains that theories of psychosomatic illness must shift, as we uncover ever more scientific research validating that consciousness is a body-mind phenomenon.

6

The New Science of Psychoneuroimmunology:
Everything Is Psychosomatic

As a groundbreaking neuroscientist, Pert's research helped to create the foundation for an entirely new interdisciplinary branch of science called "Psychoneuroimmunology" or PNI. PNI unites the three classically separated sciences of neuroscience, immunology, and endocrinology, and the associated glands, and organs into a multidirectional communication network, linked by information carrying molecules called (neuro)peptides. Pert provided PNI with a clear scientific language to use, that of peptides and their receptors, also known as "information substances," thereby helping to legitimize the field. Pert notes that her preferred term was "Psychoimmunoneuroendocrinology," recognizing the inclusion of the endocrine system, but the simpler name of PNI became the accepted term in scientific circles. The more popular name for PNI soon became "mind-body medicine."

As Pert states, "Thus, we might refer to the whole system as a psychosomatic information network, linking 'psyche,' which comprises all that is of an ostensibly nonmaterial nature, such as mind, emotion, and soul, to 'soma,' which is the material world of molecules, cells, and organs. Mind and body, psyche and soma."

This space is provided for your personal and/or support group notes.
PLEASE immediately record your ideas, insights, and inspirations as they occur to you.

6

Dr. Pert's research provides scientific evidence that a biochemical basis for awareness and consciousness exists, that the mind and body are, indeed, one and that our emotions and feelings are the bridge that links the two. She explains, "The chemicals that are running our body and our brain are the same chemicals that are involved in emotion. And that says to me that we'd better pay more attention to emotions with respect to health." Using Pert's research as a foundation, we now have a new scientific understanding of the power of our minds and our feelings to directly and profoundly affect our health and well-being. This new science explains that we are one system; the brain is integrated into the body at a molecular level and, therefore, neither can be treated separately. According to Pert, our bodies are, in fact, our subconscious minds:

In the end I find I can't separate brain from body. Consciousness isn't just in the head. Nor is it a question of the power of the mind over the body... because they're flip sides of the same thing. Mind doesn't dominate body, it becomes body.

How Did Modern Medicine Get It So Wrong?

Many indigenous cultures worldwide have long been known to honor the mind/body/environment connection. Chinese medicine and East Indian Ayurveda, systems of medicine three to six thousand years old, still correlate organs and illness with specific mental/emotional states, and seek to return the patient to mind/body/spirit balance so that healing occurs organically. Even the Greek philosopher Aristotle suggested there was a connection between mood and health when he wrote, "Soul and body, I suggest, react sympathetically upon each other." So how did Western medicine come to embrace exactly the opposite view?

Blame it on Rene Descartes, a 17th century French philosopher (noted for the aphorism "I think, therefore I am") who was the personification of what we now refer to as the "Cartesian Split." Descartes needed human bodies for dissection studies and he made a deal with the Pope of his era. He would not have anything to do with the soul, the mind, or the emotions, which remained under the Church's jurisdiction. Modern medicine would take the physical body as its domain, thus dividing the human being into two separate parts that were not to overlap. Descartes declared, "Anything to do with the soul, mind or emotions, I leave to the clergy. I will only claim the realm of the body."

This space is provided for your personal and/or support group notes.
PLEASE immediately record your ideas, insights, and inspirations as they occur to you.

6

According to this paradigm, to understand the physical nature of a human being, all one had to do was take the body apart and study the various physical components (also referred to as "reductionism"). Sir Isaac Newton, the "Father of Modern Science," also maintained through his "Newtonian Construct" that only physical matter was real and that it was all that really mattered. And so the foundation was laid for the several hundred years of relating health and the curing of disease exclusively to the realm of treating the physical body. This theory is changing slowly and even today, most modern doctors will ask about physical symptoms and then prescribe drugs or surgery. Using mind to understand body is still usually labeled as "unscientific," and mind affecting body as "psychosomatic," and therefore somehow not relevant.

How Our Emotions and Thoughts Become Our Physical Body

Peptides and Receptors: The Molecules of Emotion

What exactly is a molecule of emotion? The first component is the one Pert discovered thirty some years ago that launched her scientific career—the complex molecule known as the receptor, and more specifically—the opiate receptor. She developed a method to measure it and therefore, in a backwards sort of way, prove its existence. This discovery would explain the mechanism by which such opiates as heroin or morphine create their powerful effect on the body, the mind, and the emotions. Coincidentally, Pert had a personal experience that had birthed a growing fascination about how these substances caused such a powerful effect on the body, mind, and emotions simultaneously.

After a bad fall while horseback riding, she found herself in the hospital, being given a morphine derivative to relieve the pain of a compressed lumbar vertebra. She marveled at the combination of both pain-killing effect and the mental/emotional changes induced by the drug. Pert noted the euphoria and blissful altered state she experienced every time she received an injection. She so liked the opiate's "wonderful feeling of being deeply nourished and satisfied" that she considered continuing the drug for her pain when she was released from the hospital. Although she eventually decided against that option, her intense physical and emotional experience intrigued her and she wondered about this overlap of physical and emotional effects from a single drug. In this

This space is provided for your personal and/or support group notes.
PLEASE immediately record your ideas, insights, and inspirations as they occur to you.

6

fascination she no doubt had a great deal of company. Many have wondered how such drugs as heroin, marijuana, Librium, and cocaine are able to create such intense emotional shifts. This hospital experience would later trigger an interest in proving the existence of the opiate receptor as Pert's doctoral focus.

Hundreds of thousands of receptors sit on the surface of the average cell; specialized cells such as neurons might have millions of receptors surrounding them. These receptors act as tiny scanners and sensors that wait patiently until the exact chemical key comes along that will fit into them, much like a house key is made to fit only into one specific lock. These chemical keys are called ligands and the most common of these is known as a (neuro)peptide, accounting for nearly 95% of known ligands. Pert describes what happens next as "quite amazing." The peptide delivers its chemical message to the receptor, which then transmits this message deep within the cell, triggering a chain of biochemical reactions that can create huge changes within the cell—of either a positive or negative nature.

Pert calls the peptides the second component of the molecules of emotion. She offers an analogy:

> If the cell is the engine that drives all life, then the receptors are the buttons on the control panel of that engine, and a specific peptide is the finger that pushes that button and gets things started.

Pert asked the logical question: If we all have the opiate receptor present on the surface of the cells within our bodies, then must it not follow that our bodies have the ability to make our own endogenous version of morphine? Why else would these receptors already be present on our cells? Within three years she was proven correct when the natural opiate substance manufactured within the body was discovered and eventually became known as an "endorphin," a shortened version of "endogenous morphine." The implications of this discovery are profound and suggest that we may, in fact, have a "natural pharmacopoeia" potential already present within us. Perhaps someday we will all be capable of manufacturing our own natural biochemicals at will—in effect orchestrating our own healing. According to Pert, this concept is not as farfetched as it sounds and perhaps not so far off either.

This space is provided for your personal and/or support group notes.
PLEASE immediately record your ideas, insights, and inspirations as they occur to you.

6

Implications for Disease and Healing: The Power of Unhealed Feelings

Emotions are real—they exist in time and space and are located throughout our minds and bodies. If we accept the concept that peptides and their receptors are the actual biochemicals of emotion, then their presence in the body's nervous system and nerve cells shows us that the body can be thought of as the unconscious or subconscious mind. Pert explains further:

> As investigations continue, it is becoming increasingly apparent that the role of peptides is not limited to eliciting simple and singular actions from individual cells and organ systems. Rather, peptides serve to weave the body's organs and systems into a single web that reacts to both internal and external environmental changes with complex, subtly orchestrated responses. Peptides are the sheet music containing the notes, phrases, and rhythms that allow the orchestra—your body—to play as an integrated entity. And the music that results is the tone or feeling that you experience subjectively as your emotions.

Can the kinds and numbers of emotion-linked peptides at receptor sites on our cells influence whether we will stay well or get sick? Pert suggests yes and offers the example of viral illness: "Viruses use these same receptors to enter into a cell, and depending on how much of the natural peptide for that receptor is around, the virus will have an easier or harder time getting into the cell. So our emotional state will affect whether we'll get sick from the same loading dose of a virus." This would also explain why some people get much sicker than others from an identical exposure to a virus. Pert considers, might an elevated mood of happiness, positive expectation or hope offer some protection against a virus? She answers by telling us that she has never gotten a cold while skiing—a sport she obviously loves.

What does this suggest about the process of developing disease and an individual's potential for healing? And further, what is the relationship between the mind, the emotions, and a patient's state of health? Pert believes there is a profound and direct connection:

> We are all aware of the bias built into the Western idea that the mind is totally in the head, a function of the brain. But your body is not there just

This space is provided for your personal and/or support group notes.
PLEASE immediately record your ideas, insights, and inspirations as they occur to you.

6

to carry around your head. I believe the research findings… indicate that we need to start thinking about how the mind manifests itself in various parts of the body and, beyond that, how we can bring that process into consciousness… the neuropeptides and their receptors are the substrates of the emotions, and they are in constant communication with the immune system, the mechanism through which health and disease are created.

Think of stress-related disease in terms of an information overload, a situation in which the mind-body network is so taxed by unprocessed sensory input in the form of suppressed trauma or undigested emotions that it has become bogged down and cannot flow freely, sometimes even working against itself, at cross-purposes.

Your Brain Is Not In Charge

In a July 2004 interview with New Dimensions Radio, Pert and her husband and research partner, immunologist Michael Ruff, discussed the highly complex psychosomatic communication networks of information molecules we are all made of (www.newdimensions.org). They explain that we are not "brain centric" at all and that a state of mind is, in actuality, a state of consciousness in the body as well. The origins of illness are really within us.

Our Immune Systems Can Learn and Respond

Pert tells us that neuroscience has now proved that immune cells can be conditioned to respond to stimuli, much like Pavlov's dogs were conditioned to salivate at the sound of a bell. Psychologist Robert Ader, at the University of Rochester School of Medicine, gave laboratory rats an immune-suppressing drug flavored with sweet-tasting saccharin. Eventually the rats became so conditioned to the effects that giving them only the saccharin and no drug caused their immune systems to become depressed—at the unconscious and autonomic level. Pert comments:

We know that the immune system, like the central nervous system, has memory and the capacity to learn. Thus, it could be said that intelligence is located not only in the brain but in cells that are distributed throughout the body, and that the traditional separation of mental processes, including emotions, from the body is no longer valid.

131

This space is provided for your personal and/or support group notes.
PLEASE immediately record your ideas, insights, and inspirations as they occur to you.

6

In pivotal studies at the Case Western Reserve University in Ohio, scientist Howard Hall proved that the immune system could also be conditioned consciously using self-regulatory practices such as self-hypnosis, biofeedback, guided imagery, relaxation, and autogenic training (relaxation techniques controlling physiological variables). Using several control groups, Hall demonstrated that with conscious preparation, through using one of the types of practices noted above, individuals could consciously control the stickiness of their white blood cells, as measured by both blood and saliva tests. Pert then asks the obvious question: "If the immune system can be altered by conscious intervention, what does this mean for the treatment of major diseases such as cancer?"

Can suppressing anger or other emotions contribute to the development of cancer?—a theory proposed by Dr. Lydia Temoshok later in this Report. Since expressing emotions contributes to a free flowing network of peptides and cellular communication in the body, Dr. Pert says:

> *Absolutely. My research has shown me that when emotions are expressed... all systems are united and made whole. When emotions are repressed, denied, not allowed to be whatever they may be, our network pathways get blocked, stopping the flow of the vital feel-good unifying chemicals that run both our biology and our behavior.*

A general theory of cancer suggests that we all have errant or mutated cancer cells created in our bodies every day, yet only some individuals will go on to develop the disease. Normally our immune systems destroy these errant cells, yet in individuals whose immune systems are severely compromised, this mechanism fails. If the immune system is influenced by the "molecules of emotion" and the peptide/receptor system in the body, then what happens if the free flow of peptides is interrupted on a continual basis by the repressed emotions? Pert says it is not too hard to figure out what might happen in such a case:

> *To repress these emotions and not let them flow freely is to set up a "disintegrity" in the system, causing it to act at cross-purposes rather than as a unified whole. The stress this creates, which takes the form of blockages and insufficient flow of peptide signals to maintain function at*

This space is provided for your personal and/or support group notes.
PLEASE immediately record your ideas, insights, and inspirations as they occur to you.

6

the cellular level, is what sets up the weakened conditions that can lead to disease.

Health is not just a matter of thinking "happy thoughts." Sometimes the biggest impetus to healing can come from jump-starting the immune system with a burst of long-repressed anger. How and where it's expressed is up to you—in a room by yourself, in a group therapy situation where the group dynamic can often facilitate the expression of long-buried feelings, or in a spontaneous exchange with a family member or friend. The key is to express it (appropriately) and then let it go, so that it doesn't fester, or build, or escalate out of control.

How to Use This Information to Heal:
Dr. Candace Pert's Eight-Part Program

In her trailblazing book, Pert suggests a program of eight ways to stay healthy, or to heal if a disease state is already present. The foundational concept for all that follows is to acknowledge and claim all your feelings because they are the entrance point into the bodymind's communication network.

6

1) Become conscious. Educate yourself about these processes and become aware of how your bodymind operates to maintain wellness.

2) Learn to access the Psychosomatic Network in order to enter the bodymind's conversation and redirect it when necessary. Use an awareness of the past experiences and conditioning stored in the receptors on your cells, to release them at an emotional level. Help for this process can include psychotherapy, personal growth seminars, guided visualization, meditation, hypnotherapy, prayer, etc.

3) Explore your dreams. Dreams are one of the bodymind's methods of exchanging information for growth and healing.

   Capturing that dream and re-experiencing the emotions can be very healing, as you either integrate the information for growth or decide to take actions toward forgiveness and letting go... your dreams relate not just to your mind, but to your body as well. Dreams can be your own

This space is provided for your personal and/or support group notes.
PLEASE immediately record your ideas, insights, and inspirations as they occur to you.

6

early-warning system, letting you know if a medical condition is developing, and helping to bring your attention to the problem area. The body may be discussing this condition with the mind, and you can get in on the conversation by consciously recalling the dream... once you make the decision to pay attention to your dreams, they will start to speak to you, and you will understand them with ever-greater fluency over time, with practice.

4) Get in touch with your body. "Your body is your subconscious mind and you can't heal it by talk alone." We can access our minds and our emotions through the physical body. Use bodywork or movement therapy to heal stuck emotions. Take a walk, run, have a massage or spinal adjustment, get a few hugs, and see how you feel. Using touch and massage, physical manipulation of various types can release stored or blocked emotions by clearing internal pathways. Many healers or practitioners of Eastern healing systems can see blocked energy in the body and are trained to release it at a physical level. All injuries and traumas are stored in the tissues of the body. Pert concludes, "... almost every other culture but ours recognizes the role played by some kind of emotional catharsis or energy release in healing."

5) Reduce stress. In Pert's opinion, the most effective way to reduce stress is to learn to meditate and practice it regularly.

6) Exercise. Modern lifestyles encourage a sedentary life-style. The body was made for moving. Pert suggests trying yoga.

7) Eat wisely. "Eating, because of its survival value, has been widely interpreted by evolution to be a highly emotional event." Our gastro-intestinal tracts are densely lined with peptides and receptors that busily process information rife with emotional content. Here is also where our "gut feelings" happen.

8) Avoid substance abuse. These addictive substances bind to our receptors, blocking the natural flow of our own peptides. For example, alcohol binds to what is known as the GABA receptor. Using alcohol to excess floods our GABA receptors, eventually causing them to decrease in sensitivity and/or number, making recovery more difficult over time. This same kind of action applies to marijuana, tobacco, cocaine, and even sugar.

This space is provided for your personal and/or support group notes.
PLEASE immediately record your ideas, insights, and inspirations as they occur to you.

6

If we can learn to communicate with our bodyminds, we can tap into our body's own language to better understand and facilitate healing. Pert has come to believe that emotions are the key to coordinating all the parts of us into a harmonious and healthy whole.

New Paradigm Medicine: Health Care of the Future

In November 2002, Dr. Pert and her research partner, Dr. Michael Ruff, were honored for their scientific contributions by The National Foundation for Alternative Medicine at an awards ceremony in Washington, DC. They were asked to submit a summary of their views about the future of health care. Excerpts from this summary are provided below. Pert calls this view "New Paradigm Medicine."

We have coined the phrase "New Paradigm Medicine" to reflect the fact that it uses the established scientific method and will require quantum physics to understand the scientific under-pinnings. The terms alternative, integrative, and complementary are political, not scientific terms. We believe that New Paradigm Medicine will be fully scientifically validated one day.

… We are not a collection of separate organs or systems, but an information network in which our cells are constantly moving from one location to another as they are being formed or replaced, regulated by the molecules of emotion.

… Thus cancer, in particular, will be appreciated as a disease of the mind as well as the body and treated at centers… where body, mind, and spirit are considered. One day, cancer will be cured by interventions that release emotions in a controlled fashion such as guided imagery, art therapy, animal therapy, massage and bodywork, neurolinguistic programming, energy psychology, chiropractic, and, last but not least, music therapy. These will be used in combination—"cocktails"—scientifically optimized and validated protocols by skilled practitioners, and will actually cure or prolong high quality life in many cancers.

Whatever the pain, it's actually the brain where it is perceived. Sophisticated biofeedback methods instead of drugs or surgery will be used to treat it more successfully, along with the methods above—and more.

6

This space is provided for your personal and/or support group notes.
PLEASE immediately record your ideas, insights, and inspirations as they occur to you.

6

Nutrition will be taken extremely seriously. The fact that most of today's crops are grown for appearance and are seriously depleted of essential nutrients will be appreciated, and supplements and superfoods will be used, based upon controlled scientific clinical data.

The Spiritual Connection

Pert was one of the scientific experts interviewed in the highly acclaimed Bill Moyers PBS series, "Healing and the Mind." At one point, she asked Moyers, "Can we account for all human phenomena in terms of chemicals? I personally think we're going to have to bring in that extra-energy realm, the realm of spirit and soul that Descartes kicked out of Western scientific thought."

She describes this spiritual viewpoint in her book as well:

Yes, we all have a biochemical psychosomatic network run by intelligence, an intelligence that has no bounds and that is not owned by any individual but shared among all of us in a bigger network, the macrocosm to our microcosm, the "big psychosomatic network in the sky." And in this greater network of all humanity, all life, we are each of us an individual nodal point, each an access point into a larger intelligence. It is this shared connection that gives us our most profound sense of spirituality, making us feel connected, whole. As above, so below.

Words of Wisdom: Aim for Emotional Wholeness

Pert concludes her book with the following simple recommendations, gleaned from all the scientific data used in describing the tenets of Psychoneuroimmunology and their implications for healing:

Aim for emotional wholeness. When you're upset or feeling sick, try to get to the bottom of your feelings. Figure out what's really eating you. Always tell the truth to yourself. Find appropriate, satisfying ways to express your emotions. And if such a prescription seems too challenging, seek professional help to feel better. I believe the alternative or complementary therapies are a form of professional help much less likely to do harm and more likely to do good than conventional approaches. They work by shifting our natural balance of internal chemicals around, so we

This space is provided for your personal and/or support group notes.
PLEASE immediately record your ideas, insights, and inspirations as they occur to you.

6

can feel as good as possible. They are often particularly helpful for alleviation of the many chronic maladies that currently have no good medical solutions....

Last but definitely not least, health is much more than the absence of illness. Live in an unselfish way that promotes a state of spiritual bliss that truly helps to prevent illness. Wellness is trusting in the ability and desire of your bodymind to heal and improve itself, if given half a chance. Take responsibility for your own health—and illness.

What the Bleep Do We Know?

If you would like to know more about the science behind how our thoughts and emotions create our reality, including our state of health, then you should consider seeing the film "What the Bleep Do We Know!?" This is a pioneering, user-friendly documentary/movie that uses entertaining visual effects and story-telling to demonstrate the tenets of quantum physics and mind-body science as the force behind the creation of our daily lives. Interviews with award-winning physicists and other researchers and scientists, including Candace Pert, are woven provocatively throughout the movie. See www.whatthebleep.com for more information or for ordering DVD's.

Current Research and Publications

Candace Pert is the author of *Molecules of Emotion: The Science Behind Mind-Body Medicine* and "Your Body is Your Subconscious Mind," a two-cassette tape set. Dr. Pert and her research partner, Dr. Michael Ruff, have published over two hundred fifty scientific articles on peptides and their receptors and the role of these neuropeptides in the immune system. They hold a number of patents for modified peptides in the treatment of psoriasis, Alzheimer's, chronic fatigue syndrome, stroke, and head trauma. One of these, peptide T, is currently in Phase II trials in the U.S. for the treatment of AIDS and neuroAIDS.

Contact Information

Professor, Department of Physiology & Biophysics
Georgetown University School of Medicine, Washington, DC

This space is provided for your personal and/or support group notes.
PLEASE immediately record your ideas, insights, and inspirations as they occur to you.

7

CHAPTER 7

Do You Have a Cancer Personality?:
Lydia Temoshok, PhD

Director of The Behavioral Medicine Program, Biotechnology Institute,
University of Maryland Medical School

*"I've described the experience of cancer as a crossroads in your life,
when you're confronted with both danger—and opportunity.... What
changes you make turn this experience from what (at first) may seem like
a prison sentence into an opportunity for healing and a better life."*

—Lydia Temoshok,
Co-Author, *The Type C Connection: The Mind-Body Link to Cancer and
Your Health*

Unraveling the "Type C" Connection:
Implications for Prevention and Recovery

Can our emotions and behavior affect our risk of getting cancer, or our recovery
from this disease? This is the question Dr. Temoshok was asked to consider in
1979 when she agreed to begin an intriguing and controversial research study
with melanoma patients. Richard Sagebiel, MD, head of the Melanoma Clinic
at the University of California at San Francisco, had begun to notice "a strange
pattern of stress and coping" common to most of his patients. He thought this
might be a significant factor in the connection between cancer and behavior.
He contacted Temoshok to discuss the potential for a formal research study.

Temoshok had already been studying the effects of stress on health while on
staff at the University of California School of Medicine. She is a psychologist
nationally recognized in the fields of behavioral medicine, psychosocial oncology, and HIV/AIDS research. Temoshok started spending time at the Melanoma
Clinic, interviewing patients, and conducting a preliminary investigation. What
she found was so exciting and ripe with potential for changing the develop-

This space is provided for your personal and/or support group notes.
PLEASE immediately record your ideas, insights, and inspirations as they occur to you.

7

ment and treatment outcome of this dreaded disease that she made the decision to devote all her time to the study of the psychology of cancer patients.

What Temoshok found in interviewing these one-hundred fifty patients was a striking and amazingly similar pattern of behaviors. These melanoma patients were overwhelmingly nice. Yes, they were excessively nice, pleasant to a fault, uncomplaining, and unassertive. They went far out of their way and changed their schedules to make time to talk with her—so as not to disappoint her. The patients seemed extremely worried about their disease progression—but not for themselves. They worried about the effect it was having on their families: "I'm fine, but I'm really worried about my husband. He takes things so hard…."

Describing the Type C Behavior Pattern

In effect, the melanoma patients were using a form of denial as a coping strategy. Temoshok began to suspect that there was much more than simple denial at work and she soon began to recognize a common pattern. These patients were "pleasers" who had spent their entire lives trying to be accepted by others—spouses, parents, siblings, co-workers, friends, etc. Their very identities seemed to be derived from how they were perceived by others in their lives. Temoshok described these patients in this way: "Out of touch with their primary needs and emotions, they look to others for signals on how to think, feel, and act." She named this set of behavior traits and coping methods the "Type C" phenomenon, and she developed her theories from psychological, social, and biological perspectives.

> …What they shared was a manner of handling life stress. The melanoma patients coped by keeping their feelings under wraps. They never expressed anger, and rarely did they acknowledge fear and sadness. They maintained a façade of pleasantness even under the most painful or aggravating circumstances. They strived excessively to please people they cared about, to please authority figures, even to please strangers.

Temoshok devised a series of scientific studies to explore Type C behavior patterns and found a strong correlation with the development and progression of cancer—though by no means was this a simple case of cause and effect. There are many risk factors for developing cancer. However, Temoshok did uncover a profound relationship between repressed emotions and the depression of the

This space is provided for your personal and/or support group notes.
PLEASE immediately record your ideas, insights, and inspirations as they occur to you.

7

immune system—our first line of defense against cancer.

> *Type C behavior is an extreme version of coping methods many of us employ—we appease others, deny our true feelings, and conform to social standards. But my study of the melanoma patients led me to convincing evidence that our physical health is compromised when we chronically repress our needs and feelings to accommodate others. I was able to find evidence that this coping style weakens our immune defenses and leaves us more vulnerable to cancer progression.*

The landmark book *Type A Behavior and Your Heart* (by Meyer Friedman and Ray H. Rosenman, 1974) had already identified the Type A behavior pattern and its connection to the development of heart disease. Those exhibiting Type A behavior patterns are almost pathologically impatient, highly charged and competitive, filled with anger and hostility that they express freely, and are consistently focused on their own needs. Now for the first time its polar opposite, the Type C behavior pattern, was identified and correlated with immune dysfunction and the development and progression of cancer. Temoshok points out that most healthy people lie somewhere in the middle between these two polarities of Type A and Type C. This healthy middle ground is sometimes identified as the Type B pattern.

It is not whether we have stress—for surely we all have many highly stressful factors in our lives. Rather it is how we cope with these stressful circumstances that is a determining factor in the state of our health. Temoshok summarizes this concept: "Stress per se is not a critical factor in illness—it's the strength or weakness of one's coping mechanism."

After extensive psychological testing and interviews, Temoshok identified strong Type C patterns in at least three-quarters of the one-hundred fifty melanoma patients she studied. Type C actually refers less to their personality than to the behavior pattern they used to cope with outer stress and inner distress. She found that these patients exhibited most or all of the following behaviors:

♦ They did not express, and were often unaware of, any feelings of anger, past or present.

♦ They tended not to experience or express any other negative emotions such as fear, anxiety, or sadness.

This space is provided for your personal and/or support group notes.
PLEASE immediately record your ideas, insights, and inspirations as they occur to you.

7

- They were patient, unassertive, cooperative, and appeasing with work, social and family relationships, and also compliant with external authority.

- They were overly concerned with meeting others' needs and insufficiently engaged in meeting their own needs. They were often self-sacrificing to an extreme.

She also observed and scientifically verified the following facts:

- Patients who were more emotionally expressive had thinner tumors and more slowly dividing cancer cells, and a much higher number of lympho-cytes (immune cells) invading the tumor.

- Patients who were less emotionally expressive had thicker tumors and more rapidly dividing cancer cells, with far fewer lymphocytes invading the tumor.

Avoiding Self-Blame and Guilt

7

Clearly not wishing to encourage cancer patients to blame themselves for bringing on their cancers, Temoshok spends an entire chapter in her book explaining how using a "compassionate self-awareness of Type C behavior" can help patients rise above self-blame or victim behavior… as they are noto-riously prone to guilt and self-blame already. Knowledge is power, however, and using this information to shift self-destructive behavior patterns can make the all-important difference between surviving and dying. Most of us use cop-ing mechanisms we developed in childhood to survive life's inevitable traumas. Recognizing where these patterns no longer serve us and are, in fact, hurting us, provides the first step to a transformed life on many levels.

I also learned that people did not bring cancer on themselves. Their Type C behavior began unwittingly and persisted without conscious volition. No one can be blamed for mind-body factors in cancer, because no one intentionally develops the cancer-prone behavior pattern. Furthermore, without knowledge of the Type C cancer link, how could someone realize that his behavior might impact his cancer defense system on a molecular level?

This space is provided for your personal and/or support group notes.
PLEASE immediately record your ideas, insights, and inspirations as they occur to you.

7

I realized early in my research that Type C behavior had been each person's best attempt to cope with the pains, stresses, humiliations, and un-met needs of early childhood. Later in life, this coping method had liabilities—both mental and physical—that the person could become aware of and change, in order to lead a healthier and more meaningful existence. Type C behavior is associated not only with cancer but with many other diseases caused by immune dysfunction.

Temoshok has subsequently worked extensively with these theories as they relate to HIV/AIDS patients.

Repression of Anger is Common with Cancer Patients

Temoshok's identification of the repression of anger as a primary psychological defense mechanism among cancer patients is also noteworthy. She is careful to explain the difference between repression (unconscious and unaware) and suppression (knowledge of the anger, but choosing not to express it). The latter is generally not as destructive to the immune system. Is there a healthy expression of anger? Temoshok quotes *Love is... Everything* author Stephen Levine, who describes healthy anger as having "the quality of an unwillingness to allow things to remain as they are." Seen in this way, anger can be used as a positive force in one's life—as an agent of constructive internal and external change—and should be expressed appropriately and released.

This type of healthy anger should not be confused with resentment that can fester beneath the surface for long periods of time and literally eat away at us. Temoshok reflects on the importance of forgiveness in the following statement: "We must evaluate the contribution that factors such as forgiveness may have on health—both across the board and for those already afflicted with serious and chronic life-threatening conditions." Some people will need to take time to process and express old angers and resentments, while some (like Greg Anderson, in chapter 11 of this Report) will be able to make the leap directly into forgiveness and release. Do not judge yourself if this is a slow and difficult process. Just keep moving through it.

This space is provided for your personal and/or support group notes.
PLEASE immediately record your ideas, insights, and inspirations as they occur to you.

7

How Type C Behavior Patterns Contribute to Cancer

Temoshok devotes part of her book, *The Type C Connection: The Mind-Body Link to Cancer and Your Health* (1993), to a discussion of the science behind how mind, emotions, and body interact on a physiological level to cause disease. She notes, "The answers are beginning to be understood, in the wake of a veritable scientific revolution in the study of psyche and soma." Candace Pert (covered in this Report) published her groundbreaking book, *Molecules of Emotion,* four years later in 1997—demonstrating scientifically and dramatically, for the first time, the complex neuropeptide system and the actual process through which our emotions create actual physiological changes in our cells and organs. These changes can be health promoting or health limiting. Temoshok says:

> *Our entire view of health and illness is undergoing a seismic change. The strongest wave of change is the recognition that mind-body relationships can have a profound effect on our state of health or disease. A new science, Psychoneuroimmunology, is charting a labyrinth of mind-body connections involving brain structures, chemical messengers, and immune cells. Researchers in this young field are discovering that how we think and feel alters the strength of our immune system, the body's network of defense against disease.*

7

This is empowering information, indeed, because it helps us understand which behaviors and ingrained patterns we can begin to change in order to strengthen our immune systems, to allow our bodies to organically prevent disease, and to help heal ourselves when imbalances (diseases) are already present.

You Can Transform Your Type C Behavior and Begin to Heal

Temoshok also outlines processes to shift Type C behavior patterns. She calls it: Type C: Transformation for Recovery. The book includes stories of patients she has worked with and the profound effect that even small shifts of the Type C patterns had on the course of their disease. The basics of the Type C transformation process include nine goals tailored specifically for cancer patients:

This space is provided for your personal and/or support group notes.
PLEASE immediately record your ideas, insights, and inspirations as they occur to you.

7

1) To develop awareness of your needs

2) To discover your inner guide

3) To reframe your ideas about your feelings

4) To learn the skills of emotional expression with doctors, nurses, friends, and family members

5) To take charge of your medical care

6) To get the social support you need

7) To secure your legitimate rights

8) To work through hopelessness

9) To cultivate a fighting spirit

One way to describe your therapeutic goal to prospective counselors is that you want to transform every part of your coping style that might create a dysfunction or a weakening of your immune defenses and thereby make you more vulnerable to disease development or progression. Finding the right professional help to shift Type C behavior patterns is tantamount to survival in many cases. It is important to discover which type of psychotherapy or other therapeutic approach works best for you. These can include supportive-expressive and psychospiritual counseling, hypnotherapy, meditation, visualization, dreamwork, energy balancing techniques, art and music therapies, biofeedback, many kinds of bodywork, and more. There are mind-body techniques available in most alternative, complementary or integrative clinics.

Temoshok offers the following affirmation for cancer patients to use to reinforce these nine goals. If you recognize yourself in some of the characteristics of the Type C pattern, you may want to write out this short narrative and read it daily. Remember: small steps and small victories accumulate over time to get you where you want to ultimately be. Celebrate each one.

This space is provided for your personal and/or support group notes.
PLEASE immediately record your ideas, insights, and inspirations as they occur to you.

7

My mind and body need as much rest and relaxation as possible. In order to get well, I must pay attention to my needs above all else. This may seem self-centered, but I know that I'm a very giving person—I have been my whole life—and now I need to be indulged a bit. I have to take care of myself so that I have the best chance for recovery. If I try to be courageous at all times and strong for other people, I'll be falling back into my old pattern. I realize now that it's depleting to play that role.

I'm optimistic about getting well but I can't simply rid myself of all negative thoughts. I'm going to give myself permission to be sad, grumpy, and scared. I find it a great relief to allow these feelings to come out with other people—it was a strain to hide them all the time. I want to be a "good patient," but I can no longer live up to the label "perfect patient." I'm going to take as much time as I need to get well. These are gifts I'm giving myself, and they make me feel good about myself and my recovery.

Dr. Lawrence LeShan, a leading cancer psychotherapist and a recognized pioneer in the field of Psychoneuroimmunology, describes these same concepts in chapter 5. He states that each of us must develop "a fierce and tender concern for all parts of ourselves so that no part of our being is left standing outside the door, whimpering: 'Is there nothing for me?' Too many people feel undervalued and unworthy. How many times have we allowed societal messages or our own negatively-programmed minds to override our inner voice, the truth of our being?"

This is the beginning of the Type C transformation and the shift toward embracing all of our parts, including our "shadows," and unleashing the healing potential we all carry within us.

Dr. Temoshok's book with co-author Henry Dreher contains many encouraging success stories about cancer patients who used these theories and techniques with inspiring and profound results. The book is currently out of print; however, there are used copies available through Amazon.com and other booksellers.

This space is provided for your personal and/or support group notes.
PLEASE immediately record your ideas, insights, and inspirations as they occur to you.

8

CHAPTER 8

Creating Recovery:
Optimum Health Institute

[Note from Cynthia: I first learned about Optimum Health Institute (OHI) from an exceptional cancer survivor who was part of the Education Advisory Committee at the National Foundation for Alternative Medicine. OHI was the first stop on her healing journey, where she stabilized and began to heal her late stage IV pancreatic cancer. She returns at least once a year and whole-heartedly recommends it to others who ask how she created her miracle of healing. Based on her endorsement, I visited OHI, San Diego, two years ago. I was impressed with the quality of the classes, the enthusiastic and caring staff, and the incredible value OHI represents for very ill individuals who definitely require a multi-week stay. At OHI, many who would not normally be able to afford a residential healing program have the opportunity to participate. I came away wishing there were more OHI's around the country so many more people could use them on a regular basis.]

A Serious Health-Building Life-style Program
Embracing Body, Mind, and Spirit

The Optimum Health Institute has a very simple philosophy that it communicates clearly throughout all components of the program: the body is a self-cleansing, self-healing organism when it is given the proper tools with which to work. These tools include a raw organic diet, freshly juiced wheatgrass, maximum fluid intake, exercise to encourage lymphatic drainage and energy movement, colon cleansing, and the detoxification of mind and emotions. The Institute strongly emphasizes the need for mental and emotional detoxification as key components for optimal healing and wellness.

OHI promotes whole-person healing, and the program emphasizes self-discipline and the value of taking responsibility for oneself. This is not suggested to be a

This space is provided for your personal and/or support group notes.
PLEASE immediately record your ideas, insights, and inspirations as they occur to you.

8

"quick fix" solution to chronic or degenerative illness. A three to six month commitment to this type of whole-person protocol is normally minimal in order for deep changes in the body and mind to manifest and stabilize.

There are no medical personnel at OHI, because this program does not provide medical treatments, health evaluations or recommendations. All persons follow approximately the same standard diet and detoxification program, and are responsible for their own care while participating. Since this is not a treatment protocol but a natural health-building life-style program, many different diseases and stages of wellness are present in those participating in the program. No discussion of type of illness is ever mentioned in the registration process; in fact, it is requested during orientation that reasons for being at the Institute not be discussed with others. OHI teaches that there are no diseases, simply different "health opportunities."

"Healing circles," generally only taking three to five minutes or so, are held before every meal, creating a real sense of community among guests. The feeling of connection from being in a supportive and caring community is, no doubt, also an important part of the healing process.

The Optimum Health Institute is a non-profit organization and a non-denominational mission of the Free Sacred Trinity Church, based on the ancient Essene tradition. Do not let the term "church" mislead you; this is not a religious program in the least, and even the spiritual aspects are made more acceptable by the substitution of certain phrases and words, such as the term "alpha technique" rather than meditation. OHI sees its mission as helping people reconnect with their "Source," no matter how they view that Source.

8

An Interview with One of OHI's Founders: Pam Nees

Pam has been at Optimum Health Institute since its inception in 1976 and she is now the last surviving founder. In its twenty-nine years of operation, she notes that approximately 75,000 individuals have visited the Institute and been transformed in some way. She emphasized that visitors are definitely not "patients" and are treated as valued "guests."

Pam feels strongly that self-responsibility is integral to the success people achieve: "We are responsible and accountable to every cell in our bodies for

This space is provided for your personal and/or support group notes.
PLEASE immediately record your ideas, insights, and inspirations as they occur to you.

8

the choices we make." She describes many guests as arriving "fragmented" and out of balance. "What OHI tries to do," she explained, "is to try to pull the pieces back together again, to integrate each of them back into a truly 'wholistic' being." Over the years, she has witnessed many miraculous results in healing the hearts, minds, and bodies of visitors. Of course, the physical healing is always the most obvious and dramatic, but the mental, emotional, and spiritual healing happens just as often. Pam remarked that the OHI protocol is so "low-tech" that people cannot believe the results can be as profound as they are. She continued, "It's so simple, people don't believe it can really work." But it does, sometimes in ways that are nothing short of magical.

Interestingly, in agreement with other discussions within this Report, Pam noted that she has observed the same pattern of a very stressful or traumatic event occurring eighteen to twenty-four months before disease manifests in an individual. She often asks guests what was happening in their lives during this time period to get them to think about this. She has also observed the extremely high levels of stress many people are dealing with in today's world and how OHI attempts to teach them how to lessen its impact or release much it.

Pam explained that since there are no healthcare professionals on staff, guests are required to be in contact with their own doctors or other healthcare providers while at OHI. This is because of the rapid body changes that occur during serious detoxification. She noted that the need for prescription medication is diminished very quickly and typically dosages should be reduced, sometimes significantly.

Key to Life-style Changes and Healing:
OHI's 40 Classes Each Week

The Optimum Health Institute recognizes the importance of educating guests in how to change their lives, lessen stress, embrace a healthier diet, detox their bodies, balance their emotions, and attain more positive mental attitudes. For this, they offer forty classes every week: of the forty, fourteen are directly concerned with mental, emotional, and spiritual healing; the rest are related to diet, instruction in food preparation, physical detoxification, and exercise. Some courses include "Your Life is a Gift," "Mind/Body Connection," "Advanced Alpha Technique," "Emotional Detoxification," "Mental Detoxification," *"You*

This space is provided for your personal and/or support group notes.
PLEASE immediately record your ideas, insights, and inspirations as they occur to you.

8

Validation," "Self Esteem." A group toning class is especially powerful.

There is also a formal "Release Ceremony" held each week. All who wish to let go of anything in their lives (such as illness, relationship, job) write the message on paper and then all the papers are burned together—quite a powerful symbolic ritual.

The Diet and Detoxification Program

This OHI program consists of raw food, exercise, and daily enemas. There are daily classes with detailed instruction in bodily processes such as elimination and digestion. The last two weeks of the three-week program focus on teaching participants how to prepare the raw foods and create meals upon returning home. There is detailed instruction given about how to do the daily enemas (including a wheatgrass juice implant).

Daily menus typically include watermelon for breakfast; raw vegetables, sprouted seeds or grains, and fermented foods for lunch and dinner. The diet created by the late well-known health pioneer Ann Wigmore is used, including her fermented drink called Rejuvelac. The food program is kept as simple as possible and there are no sauces, dressings or salt available, although presentation is quite attractive and food amounts are more than ample. There is an optional three-day juice "fast" included in the middle of the first week of the program to give the detoxification process an extra nudge.

Raw vegetarian food creates a highly alkaline diet. Raw is used because of the belief that the natural enzymes present help digest the consumed foods quickly and easily, without additional strain on the body. This allows most of the body's available energy to be directed toward detoxification and healing. Much current nutrition-related literature refers to the very positive effect an alkalinizing diet has on many illnesses. There is also an emphasis on proper food combining, which is believed to enhance the digestive and detoxification processes.

There are workbooks, study guides, cookbooks, and videos available at the OHI store for those who wish to have this kind of support for either doing the program at home, or reviewing and reinforcing what was learned while visiting. A simple, inexpensive but well thought-out enema kit is also available for purchase in the store.

8

This space is provided for your personal and/or support group notes.
PLEASE immediately record your ideas, insights, and inspirations as they occur to you.

8

[Note from Cynthia: Many guests present during my visit had been to the Institute multiple times; there is a high return rate and very positive regard for the program. I personally met at least a dozen people who enroll once or twice every year to detox themselves and renew their dedication to wellness. One elderly gentleman present had made over seventy visits during the last twenty-six years.]

There were a variety of anecdotal stories of successful healing or improved health situations given by program participants (including cancer patients) during the regular Friday morning "Testimonials" gathering. Some of these were quite profound, including one gentleman whose massive neck tumors had softened and shrunk significantly and who was able to speak and swallow easily after three weeks. He had decided to stay for another two weeks of the program.

I was also quite surprised to learn that OHI has never paid for advertising or any kind of marketing during its twenty-nine years of providing these programs. All those who attend have discovered the Institute through word of mouth and OHI is often filled to capacity. Although the facilities are simple, many celebrities have completed the program.

Contact Information

Optimum Health Institute—San Diego
6970 Central Avenue, Lemon Grove, CA 91945
Phone: 800-993-4325

Optimum Health Institute—Austin
265 Cedar Lane, Cedar Creek, TX 87612
Phone: 512-303-4817

Website: www.optimumhealth.org

This space is provided for your personal and/or support group notes.
PLEASE immediately record your ideas, insights, and inspirations as they occur to you.

CHAPTER 9

A Life-Changing Boot Camp:
Hippocrates Health Institute

[Note from Cynthia: While at the National Foundation for Alternative Medicine, I wrote a report on Hippocrates Health Institute based on information I was given by one of our physicians who visited the Institute for an evaluation. I was very impressed with one of the statements he reported from Director Brian Clement: "30-40% of what we do here is psychological." As I have come to realize even more the importance of his statement, I knew that Hippocrates Health Institute should be included in this Report.]

Are You Ready to Love Yourself Enough to
Give Yourself Optimal Health?

When people call Hippocrates Health Institute (HHI) to ask what the Institute's "cure" rates are and what therapies will be used to cure them, they receive a response that may be eye-opening: "We do not cure you; you are responsible for your own life and your own healing. But we can help guide and support you in this." According to Clement, this approach filters out up to 90% of the people who contact Hippocrates. The remaining 10% are a courageous lot who are ready and willing to learn to heal themselves and who will submit whole-heartedly to the Institute's intensive regimen. Many seriously ill persons arrive on the Institute's doorstep as the last stop on a downhill journey of disease progression. Many are advanced cancer patients for whom conventional medicine has failed to provide a cure.

Hippocrates is a non-profit organization in Florida, founded by health pioneer Ann Wigmore and currently under the leadership of Co-Directors Brian and Anna Maria Clement. The basic protocol at Hippocrates is the "Life Change" program. If taken in its entirety, it is three weeks long and includes raw vegan food, fresh green juices (including wheatgrass juice), thirty hours of classes

171

This space is provided for your personal and/or support group notes.
PLEASE immediately record your ideas, insights, and inspirations as they occur to you.

9

weekly, blood tests, a personal health consultation with a physician, live blood cell analysis, use of exercise facilities, therapy, yoga, tai chi, chi gong, one massage weekly, and one colonic per visit. All of this is covered in the basic program cost. At additional costs are services such as spa treatments, hyperbaric oxygen, I.V. treatments and private psychotherapy apart from the group sessions that are offered. Nevertheless, the basic program is complete and, when fully embraced, is all one needs for beginning the healing journey.

The program cost also includes lifetime counseling by either email or fax.

An Interview with Co-Director Brian Clement

We spoke with Brian about the Hippocrates philosophy and Life Change program. He has been involved in the natural health movement for thirty-five years, the last eighteen at Hippocrates in his current position as Co-Director with his wife, Anna Maria (also a very experienced health educator who was formerly in charge of the largest natural health facility in Sweden). Brian is a much sought-after lecturer worldwide and has spent a great deal of time researching natural methods of healing with international scientists, physicians and clinics. He travels up to two months a year lecturing and studying.

Of greatest interest for this Report was Brian's explanation of the Institute's focus on mental and emotional balance. He began with a very powerful statement: "I am 100% clear that ALL healing requires the psychological aspects to be dealt with. I cannot get people to do this program unless they like themselves, love themselves, unless they know who they are and where in life they're going. This can only be sparked through emotional work and a change in mental attitude." Brian even went so far as to offer, "If you did everything perfect physically, followed the perfect diet, and you did not address the mental and emotional aspects of an illness, you would not make it. You might live longer and suffer less, but you wouldn't make it." These are strong words coming from someone who has worked with thousands of very sick people over several decades.

Based on that level of understanding, the Institute has a staff of three psychotherapists, all with different backgrounds and styles. Brian has structured it this way so that he can match the different personalities of guests with an appropriate

9

This space is provided for your personal and/or support group notes.
PLEASE immediately record your ideas, insights, and inspirations as they occur to you.

9

counseling style and recommend the right therapist when he feels a particular guest needs individual help—something that happens quite often. For example, some guests will do better with a strong, direct therapeutic style; some with a softer more pastoral style; and some may prefer to work with a therapist who has been in their shoes, has healed from a long-term chronic disease, and is now committed to helping others. Brian noted that approximately 50-70% of all guests see a therapist privately during their visit—this is strongly encouraged as integral to the healing experience.

Brian also offered an interesting metaphor for the human journey that he shares with guests. It portrays humanity as a sailboat on the sea of life. Making up the structure of the boat are the physical aspects of life and good health, such as food, exercise, shelter. The water surrounding the boat represents the emotions. Depending upon our personal perception, the waters can be calm or stormy and can take the form of a pond, a lake, a river or an ocean. Finally, the wind that fills our sails is the spiritual aspect of life.

Nutrition

The fundamental philosophy of Hippocrates is based on the diet and detoxification program developed by Ann Wigmore. Over the years the Life Change program has evolved into its present form described by the Institute as the definitive blueprint for people's transitions into a healthier life-style.

The nutrition program is referred to as a "New Era of HOPE." HOPE refers to Hormones, Oxygen, Phytochemicals and Enzymes: all-important constituents of the vegan raw diet that create an ideal chemistry within the body for healing disease and enhancing wellness.

Classes

The following subjects, taught within the thirty hours of weekly classes, relate directly to mental and emotional issues: Internal Awareness, Psychoneuro-immunology, Stress Management, Visualization and Positive Thinking, The Root Cause of Disease, Exploring Body Messages, the Healing Circle, and others.

Brian also explained that his lectures, even when they concern physical body topics, are often integrated with mental and emotional perspectives. The Clement team teaches many of the classes themselves. A complete list of classes is on the Institute's website.

This space is provided for your personal and/or support group notes.
PLEASE immediately record your ideas, insights, and inspirations as they occur to you.

9

Health Educator Program

Health Educator Certification Programs are offered three times per year. The schedule is nine weeks for new students and six weeks for alumni who have already completed the three-week Life Change program. This is an intensive exploration of the Living Foods Life-style. Students not only "walk the walk" and "talk the talk," but also experience detoxification and recharging on physical, emotional, mental and spiritual levels. They explore and expand perceptions of themselves as individuals worthy of actualizing personal life goals and leave the course with the confidence, clarity and focus to create abundance and joy in their lives and the lives of others.

Classes include: Art Therapy, Herbology, Neuro-Linguistic Programming, Massage Therapy, The History of Living Foods, Positive Thinking, Enzymatic Nutrition, Anatomy and Physiology. All courses provide regeneration and balance for the body, emotions, and mind.

The course can be attended by healthcare providers—or anyone who wants to improve personal health or help family and friends. Since its inception, the Health Educator Program has graduated students from twenty-five countries.

Staff

9

Andy Bernay-Roman, RN, MS, LMHC is one of the Hippocrates psychotherapists (his work will be discussed in the next chapter of this Report). Andy has written *Deep Feeling, Deep Healing: The Heart, Mind and Soul of Getting Well*, a book that includes many stories about how he works with guests at Hippocrates. The other primary therapist is a licensed mental health counselor and licensed clinical social worker who has masters degrees in both philosophy and theology. These therapists are extraordinary resources for guests to address the mental and emotional causes underlying much chronic disease.

Private Mind/Body Psychotherapy sessions are offered at Hippocrates. These sessions are based on the theories of Psychoneuroimmunology and are described as "drawing on various deep-feeling and body-focused techniques, as appropriate for your situation. Unlock and safely release painful memories, catastrophic conclusions of childhood and unexpressed emotions. Empower

This space is provided for your personal and/or support group notes.
PLEASE immediately record your ideas, insights, and inspirations as they occur to you.

9

yourself with new life-affirming choices."

There is also a board-certified oncologist on staff for many seriously ill guests who seek out Hippocrates in the late stages of their disease. This Institute differs from Optimum Health Institute (the subject of the last chapter) in this respect, as Brian explained that he and his staff feel duty-bound to provide medical care because of the large number of very sick or dying patients who seek them.

An Interview With a Breast Cancer Patient

Gayle, age forty-eight, has been to Hippocrates five times while she has worked on healing her metastatic breast cancer. At one point she had at least eighteen tumors throughout her body, including on her liver, lungs and neck. Her prognosis was bleak by conventional standards, yet she is now nearly cancer-free with only one small spot remaining on her left lung. Gayle was extremely open and enthusiastically shared her story, in the hope that it would empower other cancer patients to make the decision to take similar action and do whatever it takes to heal themselves. Her story is just one of dozens like it that have been included on the "Testimonials Board" (a bulletin board with personal stories of healing submitted by guests) at Hippocrates. Gayle estimated that there are literally hundreds of cancer patients who have come to Hippocrates and healed themselves, yet this is not a statistic the Institute can publicize, for fear of legal reprisal.

Six years ago Gayle had an extremely stressful life. Her high-pressure job required a daily commute of over two hours. She never saw her family, she was depressed and had begun to quit taking care of herself physically. When her breast cancer was diagnosed, Gayle saw an oncologist and did the conventional therapies. She then went to Hippocrates to detoxify her body, but she did very little else while there. In other words, she focused almost entirely on the physical aspects. She enrolled several more times over the ensuing years, always looking to the diet and physical therapies to keep her disease in check.

Gayle succeeded in keeping her cancer under control until being confronted with a traumatic situation with her teenage son. He began to have trouble with the law, was out of control and had to be committed to a "lockdown" type of boarding facility for rehabilitating young persons. Gayle felt she had abandoned her son and described this as one of the most painful times of her life.

This space is provided for your personal and/or support group notes.
PLEASE immediately record your ideas, insights, and inspirations as they occur to you.

9

She agonized over sending him away and then struggled with his pleas to come home. Soon after this, she found that her cancer had returned with a vengeance, with many more areas of her body now showing tumor growth— at least eighteen more tumors were counted. Her oncologist recommended chemotherapy once a week for the next six months.

At this point, Gayle returned to Hippocrates, determined to embrace the complete Life Change program 100% and to do whatever emotional work was required. She now began to do intensive psychological work with psychotherapist Andy Bernay-Roman, seeing him two or three times a week for the next six weeks. She credits this extremely difficult emotional work as probably the critical component of her success.

Gayle recognized how the loss of her mother at age six triggered major feelings of abandonment. She embraced her feelings, allowed their expression, and began to heal in a dramatic fashion. Gayle remarked how amazed she was at the level of fear that was attached to keeping her emotions suppressed. She recalled one especially powerful therapy session of emotional release when she said out loud to herself coming out of the session, exhausted but at peace, "I can breathe!"

Gayle also shared that she attended the "Healing Circles" class at Hippocrates regularly, during which Andy Bernay-Roman worked experientially with several guests as the others observed. She remarked how lucky she was to have a supportive husband, because the stories she often heard from others portrayed a very different situation. Some guests endured constant criticism and judgment from family members who continued to try to force them to make conventional choices and abandon their commitment to natural healing methods.

9

When she returned home and visited one of her oncologists, Gayle recalled, "His jaw just dropped open when he saw me. Mind you, I looked great, I was tan, I was exercising every day, I looked the picture of health. He really didn't expect to ever see me again." Her tests revealed that 97% of her cancer had now disappeared. "What did you do," he asked. "Did you go to Sloan-Kettering?" Gayle smiled and told him exactly what she had done, but he took no notes and she knew that none of this would ever be shared with another patient. She added sadly, "And I know several of his patients who were just like me…."

This space is provided for your personal and/or support group notes.
PLEASE immediately record your ideas, insights, and inspirations as they occur to you.

9

Gayle's original oncologist (not the one described in the preceding paragraph), a female physician who had decided to leave oncology for general practice, actually accompanied Gayle on her next visit to Hippocrates and participated in the program—just to find out what was producing these amazing results.

Gayle wanted to make a final point for other cancer patients. She had made the decision that she needed to completely separate herself from her normal life, to devote all her mental, emotional and physical energy to healing. During that time she made arrangements to live temporarily in California. She used email only, she took no phone calls, she put her many social and job commitments on hold, she exercised and ate raw food every day—and she ultimately discovered that almost all the tumors in her body had dissolved away in the process. Gayle said she wanted to encourage other patients to have the courage to change their lives if they needed to—no matter how difficult this would be.

The take-home lesson here is this: get a second mortgage or borrow if you must, change locations, release commitments, distance yourself from unsupportive family and friends, and find the courage to work on the mental and emotional aspects of your disease. In other words, become empowered enough to do whatever it takes to create the energy and optimal situation for recovering from your illness and healing your life.

9

Contact Information

Hippocrates Health Institute
1443 Palmdale Court, West Palm Beach, FL 33411
Phone: 561-471-8876 or 800-842-2125 (reservations only)
Email: hippocrates@worldnet.att.net
Website: www.hippocratesinst.org

This space is provided for your personal and/or support group notes.
PLEASE immediately record your ideas, insights, and inspirations as they occur to you.

10

CHAPTER 10

Jump-Start Your Healing:
Andy Bernay-Roman, RN, MS, LMHC

"Every cell in your body is eavesdropping on your thoughts."
—Deepak Chopra, MD

An innovative body-centered psychotherapist and former ICU nurse, Andy has served since 1990 as the head of the Psychological Support Department at Hippocrates Health Institute (see previous chapter). His formal training includes an emphasis on Psychoneuroimmunology. Andy teaches classes and facilitates the ongoing healing circle support group at Hippocrates as well as privately treating individuals, couples, and families. He was a 1995 nominee for the Norman Cousins Award, as well as the Rosalyn Carter Caregiver Award. Andy is the author of *Deep Feeling, Deep Healing: The Heart, Mind and Soul of Getting Well* (published in 2002; available on Andy's website or Amazon.com). He is also a certified massage therapist and licensed mental health counselor in Florida.

Andy summarized his beliefs about the ability of emotional healing to facilitate physical healing in the following quote from an article he wrote for the Hippocrates newsletter:

> *Just as important as what you eat, "what's eating you" plays a central role in the disease process, and therefore careful attention to your mental health (with a focus on feelings) is paramount to getting well. Feelings play a major role in the hierarchy of what the body can and will heal. Paying attention to feelings, especially those that may reside in repressed form within the tissues of the body, can unleash great forces for healing by normalizing hormone levels, reducing inner pressure, and generally bringing a sense of resolution to the system.... Remember, the body follows what is in the heart and mind in both illness and cure.*

10

This space is provided for your personal and/or support group notes.
PLEASE immediately record your ideas, insights, and inspirations as they occur to you.

10

During the healing circle, Andy generally works with one or two persons from the group. He hopes that during this interaction other guests will be inspired to begin their own personal journey. He teaches the Psychoneuroimmunology class, and participates in the Mind-Body Panel for guests. He described the process of healing as akin to getting into a room. There are many ways to get inside, to reach the soul. Sometimes it is through the doorway of the mind, sometimes by the heart, and sometimes via the body.

Andy remarked that there is a strong emphasis on self-responsibility at Hippocrates. This is definitely a change from conventional medicine, which tends to disempower patients. The people who come to Hippocrates are usually a select group who are highly motivated, open and willing to do whatever it takes to heal. This makes his job easier. Andy says that the mental and emotional work is integral to the healing process; "even if it's not directly causative, it gives them much more energy to use in healing.... Disease happens in our humanity, not in a vacuum."

In his book he discusses deep feelings as "the good, the bad, and the ugly":

> The first rule is to stop denying that the pain exists. Stop pretending and get real. Over and over in newly formed support groups, sessions that start out as chatty and superficial soon travel deeper towards a feeling core, delving into expressions of genuine loss, caring, and despair. The same is true of one-on-one therapy. The urge to be whole, to be real, and to feel, like a dormant seed thirsting for water, creates its own momentum, and once initiated, hopefully, carries the patient into the realm of health.

Andy describes the mechanism of mind-body healing (and of the disease process) by explaining more about how our thoughts and emotions directly influence health:

> Memory then, does not reside just in the brain. If it did, our heads would swell with experience! Memory lives throughout the body. In fact, our cells contain a perfect memory of all experiences and store it. Where do these receptor sites reside? In the soft tissues of the body, including the immune system! These information-carrying neuropeptides are the mind-body link, acting as transducers of semantic and emotional information at the cellular level. Our emotions play a role in every biochemical event that transpires within us, even while we sleep.

10

This space is provided for your personal and/or support group notes.
PLEASE immediately record your ideas, insights, and inspirations as they occur to you.

10

When our emotions trigger a cascade of brain endorphins, the natural pain killers that yield a sense of well-being, the end result is a calm, life-affirming one. When our emotions consistently trigger the release of stress hormones, designed to keep our system alert in times of emergency, the net result is life-negating and sets the stage for disease. Our emotional tone directly influences the sum total of all biochemical processes.

Treatment that ignores the central biological role of feelings cannot bring about lasting change. Mere intellectualizing doesn't cut it when it comes to imprinted repressed pain.

In his book Andy also shares a story of research on the chemistry of tears. Inducing tears of both joy and sadness in volunteers, researchers analyzed the chemical composition of each and found something remarkable: the chemistry of the tears of sadness differed significantly from the tears of joy. The only variable that could account for the difference was the change in emotions. Emotions change body chemistry. Psychiatrists use the reverse of this formula and give drugs to the physical body to change the emotions, but the direct connection between the two remains.

As an ICU nurse, Andy frequently worked with patients whose life-threatening encounters with illness "shocked them into a natural regression that often facilitated a healing. I concluded that the body WANTS to integrate at the feeling level." He described the therapeutic process as a safe atmosphere that encourages self-reflection and going within, an excursion he calls "the centropic journey":

10

Repressed feelings emerge along the way. I learned during the process that old nonintegrated feelings dominate the feeling landscape because they NEED to be integrated. They continue to color everything in the present and influence every interaction. Repressed pain robs us of our capacity for joy. Repressed sadness and anger transform into depression or some other form of inner isolation.

Andy notes that deeper work can take more time and effort than other forms of therapy "because of the defenses against pain that have kept the source of the person's problem imprinted within." He describes this process as "the Hero's Journey":

This space is provided for your personal and/or support group notes.
PLEASE immediately record your ideas, insights, and inspirations as they occur to you.

10

It involves leaving the comfortable realms of the known, crossing over the frontiers of fear and aloneness, descending into the Valley of Death itself if necessary, and ultimately returning to the surface world renewed. The psychotherapy I practice happens under the banner of such transformation and nothing less.

Andy suggests that those wishing to heal physically take the following steps in order to maintain a "clean" psychological environment:

1) *Patch up any resentments and unfinished business. Do whatever it takes so at least you know you have tried.*

2) *Make room for feelings and practice honest, appropriate expression to your present family, or to others in your relationship system. A free flow of feelings is like the healthy flow of blood in the body.*

3) *Focus on the love and appreciation you have for the other members of your system. This fosters an upward spiral of acceptance and ease in being together.*

4) *Make conscious agreements on how to handle negative emotions like anger or jealousy. A good rule of thumb about those types of feelings is that they generally do not stand alone, but overlay a deeper layer of hurt or fear. During those negative feelings, make the choice to share the whole spectrum of truth, including the more vulnerable feelings. Let yourself be vulnerable in order to cultivate trust.*

5) *Actively respect the integrity and otherness of people in your system. Avoid the traps of right and wrong. When you make someone wrong, you are literally hurting yourself.*

10

And why should we not try to rise above our negative emotions, to focus only on the positive, and relegate the negative to the recesses of our consciousness? Andy explains that negative feelings per se do not damage us, but it is in suppressing them that damage is done.

Repression infuses an anti-life message into the body... repression causes the body to cut off from certain parts, and waste energy by keeping feelings down. Reclaiming the heart by reconnecting with feelings clears a path through the jungle of human interactions and liberates us from the

This space is provided for your personal and/or support group notes.
PLEASE immediately record your ideas, insights, and inspirations as they occur to you.

10

past. Ongoing self-discovery and self-acceptance in a practical way stands as a banner that lines the road to peace and health, whereas the "get rid of it" approach ends in a tragic dead end.

As important as healthy food is to the healing process, Andy says that it takes love to create full aliveness and healing balance. He described a study of orphanages in the 1940's where the babies were well-fed, but were not held, rocked or given loving personal attention from caregivers. A unexpectedly large number of these babies simply wasted away; food and comfortable surroundings alone could not sustain them.

Beyond physical malnourishment, love deprivation stands at the root of physical and mental disease. Love deprivation can mean anything from out-and-out abuse to the less extreme situation of growing up with a particular aspect of the natural self going through life unloved, unsupported or neglected.

How to Jump-Start Your Healing Process

Andy offers thirteen principles of mind-body integration; these principles set the parameters for his type of therapy. They explain how dysfunctional and limiting patterns get wired into our systems, and also suggest how we can un-wire them. These principles are definitely worth considering within the context of the disease and healing process.

1) *What is out there goes in, and what is in there comes out.* Our nervous systems are very susceptible and absorb much of what is happening around us. Then our beliefs tend to look for evidence for backup.

2) *The system responds to stress long after the source of stress is removed* The more traumatic the stress, the more recovery time is needed.

3) *The system responds to perceived/imagined reality in the same way as it does to actual reality, and to beliefs as it does to truth.* Just the memory or reminder of a trauma can elicit a response identical to the original response.

4) *The system processes input via the laws of parsimony, or the path of least resistance, which makes the known dominate new input.* We tend to

This space is provided for your personal and/or support group notes.
PLEASE immediately record your ideas, insights, and inspirations as they occur to you.

10

understand new events based on what we already know or are already familiar with.

5) *The system maintains a record of all experiences with a triune memory, which includes body-response, emotional charge and personal meaning.*

6) *It takes effort to move from a trance state (where imprints from the past dominate experience and we cling to the familiar) to a new state.* The tendency to make the world familiar is hard-wired into us, explaining the automated or learned "knee jerk" response.

7) *The system operates on the biological imperative to avoid pain.* This is also hard-wired into us and is more intrinsic than the Freudian pleasure principle. Avoidance of pain defense mechanisms causes the conscious mind to dissociate from trauma and to fragment feeling.

8) *Experiences repressed out of consciousness remain imprinted in the system in their original form.* Painful feelings can get tucked away into unconsciousness so that we can continue functioning. Andy believes that this may explain the autoimmune response in which the body initiates an attack on the immune system as it attempts to destroy any internalized foreign matter, and feelings.

9) *The system operates on internal deductive logic.* This is not rational logic, but a loose set of associations and emotional charges. Conclusions about reality are based more on things verified by our feelings than on anything else.

10) *It takes energy to keep material repressed from consciousness.* Repression takes on-going vigilance; defenses require energy that could be used for healing.

11) *When repressed material returns to consciousness, the pain associated with it, and the energy required for the repression, does also.* All the energy required for repression now becomes available when the pain is integrated. That is very good news for physical healing.

12) *Every disintegration of experience sets integrative forces into motion.* The quest for wholeness is also hard-wired into us. The drive to become real thus has biological fuel. This is also good news.

10

This space is provided for your personal and/or support group notes.
PLEASE immediately record your ideas, insights, and inspirations as they occur to you.

10

13) Every access is a reframe. Just by accessing memories and remembering, we alter their meaning. (When we attempt to reframe without full integration of feeling, however, we end up thwarting the process of fully updating our systems. Positive thinking used as an overlay on top of painful feelings can become just another neurotic strategy to keep us from our pain.)

If the simple power of suggestion can rid a person of warts or enlarge breasts (proven facts), and the immune system can be tricked by a placebo, then surely a more thorough investigation into the deeper realm of mind and heart will uncover a veritable genie of healing.

Contact Information

Website: www.deepfeeling.com

10

This space is provided for your personal and/or support group notes.
PLEASE immediately record your ideas, insights, and inspirations as they occur to you.

CHAPTER 11

You Can Be a Cancer Conqueror:
Greg Anderson

Cancer Survivor, Author, Advocate

"When we are motivated by goals that have deep meaning, by dreams that need completion, by pure love that needs expressing, then we truly live."

—Greg Anderson

In 1984 Greg only had a few weeks to live when he made the decision to finally heal his relationships with everyone in his life, including a former "enemy." He then made a full recovery from his "incurable" late-stage metastatic lung cancer. Following his dramatic encounter with an act of forgiveness towards his former colleague, he spent considerable time alone crying in his car, finding himself incapable of driving, and completely overcome with an emotional catharsis that he had never permitted himself before. Again and again he repeated the phrase, "I'm free. I'm free. I'm free." And so he was. His physical condition began to improve from that day forward. Greg's heart, mind, and spirit had already been healed.

11

Greg's Story in His Own Words

The Law of Forgiveness is a tough taskmaster. It forces us to examine our motives. It requires us to look deep within. The work of forgiveness demands that we give up the need to always be right. That is a big request.

The Law of Forgiveness can be misunderstood. It is not asking us to betray our deepest beliefs or disregard our principles. We need not compromise our personal integrity by failing to stand up for what we hold to be true. The law does not imply that we are to live our lives trying to please everyone at the risk of being untrue to ourselves. However, the law does ask us to become keenly

This space is provided for your personal and/or support group notes.
PLEASE immediately record your ideas, insights, and inspirations as they occur to you.

11

aware of how often we engage in verbal and emotional combat that has less to do with higher principles and personal integrity than it does with our perceptions of being right.

The Law of Forgiveness demands that I come to a very important realization: in these matters, it is not my spirit that demands to be right, it is my frail ego.

Realize that this law and its demands are as true of marriages as of business transactions. Forgiveness is for the workplace and for parenting, for young and old, for black and white. Forgiveness applies to everything, to everyone, all the time. This is what is meant by life being lived most abundantly as an adventure in forgiveness.

Nothing contaminates the life of wellness more than resentment, remorse, and recrimination. These states of heart and mind do more to stand in the way of our wellness than virtually any other dynamic. If the daily practice of the Law of Forgiveness is the only way out, what does this law look like in action?

I know from vivid personal experience. I can trace the absolute turning point in my own illness directly to the work of forgiveness. Weak, emaciated, lying at home in constant pain, I was going downhill rapidly by all physical measurements. Doctors, family, even my own mind—all believed I was about to die of cancer.

Yet something kept driving me. I would place phone calls to organizations all over the country, seeking others who had gone through a similar situation and lived. I wanted to learn from their experience. I kept hearing people talk about forgiveness. "You need to forgive," said a woman in Boise, Idaho. A man from Tennessee put it plainly: "The difference is forgiveness." My first reaction was "I probably don't have many issues of forgiveness to deal with. Forgiveness isn't my problem."

I was wrong. Forgiveness was my issue. My critical attitude was first. Why did I look at a situation and always pick out what was wrong? I'd do it constantly. People were my favorite target. I would make a quick study of someone and actively seek out his Achilles' heel. "What's wrong with him?" I'd think. It was all an effort to put someone else down in order to build myself up. Distorted thinking bereft of charity and compassion.

This space is provided for your personal and/or support group notes.
PLEASE immediately record your ideas, insights, and inspirations as they occur to you.

11

The worst example was my behavior at work. When a new controller was brought in and I suddenly had to seek approval for all our division's expense budgets through this new "intruder," I saw the whole setup as a huge threat to my position. So, without really making a conscious decision, I began to attack. I became critical of the controller's plans. I tried to undermine his work. I threw stones at his policies. I became critical of him personally.

My criticism led to condemnation. I set myself up as judge and jury. If I were superior, then I was right. In fact, I always had to be right. Therefore, the new controller was, by definition, wrong. I condemned him and then went about proving it to others.

As I look back, I see that it was only three months between the time the new controller came on board and the onset of my cancer diagnosis. I believe there was a link between my toxic behavior and the onset of my illness.

What I didn't count on was a counter attack. The new controller fought back, pointing out my failures to institute more effective financial controls.

He was equally skilled at finding a person's weak point. And the battle between the two of us became a company-wide problem that began to drag everyone down.

I am saddened and mortified about how it came to a head. We were in a meeting with three other division heads and the CEO. My adversary, the controller, passed around a budget update. Trying to be flippant, I took my copy of the document, threw it across the table and proclaimed, "These numbers are a crock of __." The report hit the CEO's coffee cup, the contents of which spilled into his lap. He jumped up, glared at me, pointed a finger and said, "Get the hell out of here." I went back to my office and then headed to my car. I began to see how absolutely ludicrous my behavior had been.

That kind of behavior consumes vast amounts of emotional energy. It produces a negative and contrary spirit that is toxic to us and to others. I had my entire sense of worth invested in always being right. I suppose it was an issue of perception. I was so concerned with what other people thought of me that I never considered I might be wrong. I needed everyone to know that I was right and to acknowledge it.

11

This space is provided for your personal and/or support group notes.
PLEASE immediately record your ideas, insights, and inspirations as they occur to you.

11

But the story takes an even more bizarre twist. Within thirty days of my diagnosis of lung cancer, my adversary the controller was diagnosed with cancer. Now, I have had medical authorities tell me that he probably had been carrying the cancer for years and it had just then been discovered, as had mine. But my intuition tells me that our toxic battle contributed to the onset of both illnesses.

I underwent surgery that removed a lung. But surgery was impossible for my nemesis the controller. The disease had already spread. As the weeks passed, both of us grew progressively worse.

Four months later, a second surgery confirmed that the cancer had spread from my lung through the lymph system. The following day the surgeon made a statement that is indelibly etched in my mind. "Greg," he said, "the tiger is out of the cage. Your cancer has come roaring back. I'd give you about thirty days to live."

It was at that moment that I began my journey in search of wellness. Lying in bed, at home, I continued to deteriorate physically. But I made those phone calls in search of survivors and I kept hearing "forgive."

One morning I awoke and I realized that I did have a monumental task of forgiveness ahead of me. I felt a deep conviction that this was the thing for me to do. From my sickbed I began the solitary work of forgiveness. I believe that this was the precise turning point in my illness.

The Law of Forgiveness carries with it the idea of process. That is, there are actions and conscious decisions that are integral to the forgiveness phenomenon. Any number of legitimate ways to proceed exist, but they each share this idea of helping us release resentment, express negative feelings, and let go of past wrongs, both real and imagined. Once the idea of process has been grasped, it only needs to be applied with consistency and sincerity to bring immediate results.

The essence of the various processes is quite simple: become aware of the person toward whom we feel hostility, express active release from that hostility and picture good things happening to him or her. In the privacy of my bedroom, I made a sign on a sheet of paper.

11

This space is provided for your personal and/or support group notes.
PLEASE immediately record your ideas, insights, and inspirations as they occur to you.

11

It reads:

NAME
RELEASE
AFFIRM

With that sign propped at my bedside, I started a list of the people in my life. I put my wife first. I closed my eyes, relaxed, and created a clear picture of her in my mind. Then, from my heart, I imagined myself saying to her, "I forgive you. I totally and completely forgive you for every perceived wrong you have done—and for anything you have left undone."

And I would pause, allowing ample time to remember and release specific instances. I wouldn't dwell on the specifics. I would just recall them and release them, recognizing that it was I, not my wife, who was really being let off the hook.

I would end the work with each person by picturing something good happening to him or her. I knew that my wife wanted and needed to receive continual reassurance of my love for her. I pictured her receiving that. I knew that another person with whom I'd had a falling-out wanted a new sports car. I imagined him happily driving down the freeway in his red Porsche. The point is: part of the process I used was to actively see something good happening to the person I was forgiving.

This was not always a smooth experience. It became fascinating for me to watch my own resistance. It was relatively easy to express forgiveness and mean it. To actively release the hurt was more challenging, but repeating the release three or four times typically helped me make the emotional and spiritual shift that was required. Many times I would say, "God, you take this. I cannot handle it anymore."

The third element of the process was the real test for me. It was difficult to envision good things happening to many of the people I wanted and needed to forgive. But I was sincerely committed to the process. I did not have an expectation of ease. I would see this through.

11

This space is provided for your personal and/or support group notes.
PLEASE immediately record your ideas, insights, and inspirations as they occur to you.

11

I discovered I was intensely angry with my father. He never was able to express his love. In fact, his approach to child raising was to emotionally put down and never, not once, build up. I found it very difficult to totally release my perceptions of being wronged. And I found it next to impossible to imagine, with sincerity, something good happening to him. I spent nearly two days just on the work of forgiving my father. Tough stuff.

The work on forgiving my father taught me an important lesson. His actions resulted from huge hurts of his own. They had nothing to do with me. The inability to express love was a direct reflection of his own upbringing. I shifted my perspective from blaming him for all that was missing to understanding how I may also have contributed to the situation. I was rebellious. I did not obey. I was sarcastic. Perhaps the only way to reach me was through put-downs.

Down the list I went. Name people; forgive and release them; affirm them. Many times I went back to names, especially those where the memories created feelings of unease. And I offered my forgiveness with deep sincerity.

This insight extended to other relationships. As I would forgive and release, I still might not approve of the way a person handled a particular situation. But after completing the process of forgiveness, I could generally understand the situation better and begin to see my own part in it.

Sometimes forgiveness requires work above and beyond the call of duty. This was the case with the controller. I had spent hours forgiving and releasing and trying to imagine great things happening to him. About noon of the fourth straight day of forgiveness, I came out of the bedroom for lunch. It was then I realized that my work with him needed to take on a more personal touch. I needed to visit him and express my apologies.

This was not easy. I made a call to the office and found that he was at home and not doing well. I phoned and his wife answered. Her voice immediately telegraphed surprise and shock to be talking to me; she knew full well the battle that raged between her husband and me.

I said, "I want to come out and visit, this afternoon. When would be a good time?" She said she'd have to check. "I'll hang on," I replied. The time was set.

11

This space is provided for your personal and/or support group notes.
PLEASE immediately record your ideas, insights, and inspirations as they occur to you.

11

When was the last time your heart felt like it would pound right out of your chest? My emotions went on overdrive. On the way to his house, I wanted to turn back. My steps in making the short walk between the curb and his front door were some of the most difficult I have ever taken. The whole time, my heart was in my throat. But I pressed on. I felt that my life hinged on this sincere effort of forgiveness.

What do you say to someone whom you have previously considered an enemy? How do you communicate your changed feelings? Are words ever adequate to make up for the emotional havoc one has caused?

I was greeted and led into the bedroom, where my adversary was propped up in his bed with pillows. And with my heart pounding, adrenaline rushing, voice shaking, I barely managed to stutter out a few words to this effect:

"I have come to say I am sorry." A long pause to gather some composure. My voice still breaking, I continued: "I deeply regret the hurt I have caused you." Another pause. I remember my right hand and arm were shaking, out of my control. I tried to steady them with my left hand. In a whisper I finished: "I want you to know I wish you only the best."

Those words were imperfect, to be sure. They were delivered in a voice that was gripped with fear. But they came from my heart, sincere in every aspect. They must have been effective. Because my adversary struggled to sit up, swung his feet over the edge of the bed and motioned me to come and sit by his side.

"Greg," he said, "I am the one who needs to say I'm sorry. I'm old enough to be your father. Yet I treated you like the outcast son. Please forgive me."

His wife was crying. She knelt on the floor and the three of us embraced. We all cried. Finally, it was my old adversary who found the strength to mutter a prayer: "Dear God, forgive us all."

We said brief good-byes and I left. As I started the car back toward home, I took a deep breath and said out loud, "Whew!" A weight was being lifted. I could feel it, sense it, was part of it: the clouds that had been tormenting me were beginning to part. The day seemed brighter. Was it the sun, or was it this catharsis that had just taken place?

11

211

This space is provided for your personal and/or support group notes.
PLEASE immediately record your ideas, insights, and inspirations as they occur to you.

11

My posture changed. I went from being hunched over to sitting erect in the seat. I held my head more upright. The tension in my shoulders lessened dramatically. The wrinkles on my forehead melted away. I relaxed. The pain was gone. The quivering hand was steady. A smile came across my face. "I'm free!" I whispered. "I'm free," I repeated, this time louder. In a crescendo I exclaimed, "I'm free! I'm free! I'm free!" I shouted it: "I'm free!"

Tears gushed down my cheeks in torrents. My vision became blurred. I quickly pulled off onto a side street, parked the car and wept, out of control, for a long, long time.

I remember the eyes of a lad who came to the window. I wonder how long he had been watching me. "Hey, mister," he said, "you need help?" "No, no. I'm fine." And I made my way home.

RELEASE. SET FREE. I look back to my week of the sincere work of forgiveness and realize this was the absolute turning point in my physical healing. From that point in time, I began to gain back lost weight, manage pain more readily and hold more positive thoughts about my future.

Do I believe there was a link between this deeply spiritual work and my physical improvement? Absolutely. I believe that practicing the Law of Forgiveness changes us biochemically. And in the process, the body is released toward its optimum wellness potential.

I know that my doctor and scientist friends get very uncomfortable when I share these beliefs. But it seems we can all agree on this: life quality soars when we sincerely practice the Law of Forgiveness. And this may just be an important determinant in releasing the body's self-healing potential.

11

Life can, indeed, be lived most abundantly as an adventure in forgiveness. Forgive. Set yourself free.

This space is provided for your personal and/or support group notes.
PLEASE immediately record your ideas, insights, and inspirations as they occur to you.

11

The Cancer Recovery Foundation of America

Following his recovery from lung cancer in 1985, Greg Anderson founded what would later become The Cancer Recovery Foundation of America (CRFA), to help other cancer patients learn from what he had experienced. CRFA produces a variety of educational resources. It continues to reach out to cancer patients anywhere in the world and has expanded with branches now in Canada, Europe, and England. There are currently 254 adult cancer recovery programs internationally and 172 pediatric cancer programs. Greg has appeared on over 1,100 radio and television programs teaching his holistic recovery philosophy and techniques. There are seminars available: call CRFA at 800-238-6479 for a schedule.

Any cancer patient can call and request help. Greg's brochure, summarizing the self-described changes among six hundred of the 15,000 "terminal" cancer survivors in the CRFA database, is part of the packet of information that can be requested. It is called "Cancer: A Message to Change," and it asks the reader to consider: "What message to change is cancer asking of me?"

Greg's quest with this research was to find out if there were common characteristics of survivorship that could help others. What he found at the most basic level, underlying all of the research, was the fact that cancer survivors change—both their lives and themselves. "They create a state of body, mind, and spirit where they are well and they live from that state. Survivors heal the whole person… the changes come first; survivorship follows." These survivors were essentially asked the question: "What did you do to get well again?" Research results include summaries relating to six areas: physical, mental, social, emotional, vocational, and spiritual.

11

The following statistics seem especially relevant and important to consider:

> *One of the most common perceptions among survivors was a new and greater level of emotional awareness. 7 in 10 survivors cited emotional and psychological factors as playing a "major" role in how and when they became sick. 8 in 10 felt the same factors played a "major" role in how their immune system functioned.*

This space is provided for your personal and/or support group notes.
PLEASE immediately record your ideas, insights, and inspirations as they occur to you.

11

5 in 10 survivors cited releasing the past as a "major" factor in survivorship. This was not forgive and forget; more accurately it was forgive and learn. Survivors gave no tacit approval to abhorrent behavior from others or themselves. Rather, the focus was on detachment from hostility that freed personal energy for healing.

Greg summarized the research study with the following observation:

Personal change is pervasive among long-term cancer survivors.... By approaching cancer as a message to examine change, on as many levels of being as possible, patients make it much more likely that their healing capacities will be fully mobilized. As a bonus, quality of life improves, making it infinitely more worth living for whatever time one is given.

Extraordinary Books for Cancer Patients—
Or Anyone Who Just Wants a Better Quality of Life

A Modern-Day Parable: *The Cancer Conqueror*

Greg Anderson is the author of several remarkable books. One of his most popular, now translated into nineteen languages, is *The Cancer Conqueror,* the story of one individual's search for help and healing. It begins almost like a fairy tale: "There was once a man who had just received a diagnosis of cancer...." The truths it contains are profound and universal.

Surviving cancer is a process... and with good strategies and good physical care, whether conventional, integrative or alternative, people succeed all the time. This book is a roadmap of much of that process. Some highlights are offered here, but you can choose to learn more by ordering the book and reading it ALL (highly recommended)! It is available, along with Greg's other fine books, from CRFA.

11

Some selected highlights from *The Cancer Conqueror:*

The Cancer Conqueror encourages us to acknowledge that attitudes, beliefs, and thoughts go together to create a mental and emotional outlook toward life, an emotional lifestyle. Those emotions, either positive or negative, translate to the physical... emotions can play a central role in

This space is provided for your personal and/or support group notes.
PLEASE immediately record your ideas, insights, and inspirations as they occur to you.

11

cancer's outset and course.... Not only changed emotional states, but CHARGED emotional states. Fear. Anger. Guilt. All commonly the result of mismanaged stress. Actually the issue isn't stress, but how we manage stress.

In response to the idea that our negative attitudes and emotions contribute to our disease: The question is asked: "Does this mean I gave myself cancer?" And the answer: "Now here is the hopeful part: If you believe that you may have contributed to your illness, then you must also believe that you have the power to contribute to your recovery. The psychological and spiritual components can work either for us or against us. The choice is ours.

Let me leave you with one of Greg's favorite stories about his beliefs. One of his heroes is Christopher Columbus. At that point in history everyone believed the world was flat. But Columbus decided to challenge that belief. He took a chance, and the world has never been the same since! He was a real conqueror! Our beliefs about cancer are like that. You are a modern-day Columbus about to start a journey. Some people will tell you there is no hope, that the world is flat. Do not believe it! Instead, take a chance. Start the journey. Become a cancer conqueror!

And—become a Frog-Kisser! In continuing the "fairy-tale" feel found at times in the book, an old story with a message is adapted for cancer patients. We all remember the princess who encounters a frog who has had a spell cast over him, turning him from a handsome prince into a frog who can only be returned to his natural state with a kiss from a beautiful maiden. He tells the princess his story and asks for a kiss. She does not really feel like kissing a frog that day. It is distasteful, why should she do this? Still, she considers: "What if there really is a handsome prince under all that ugly green skin? What if he really is telling the truth? Just because I've never encountered this before doesn't mean it isn't possible. It might actually be exciting to be involved, a whole new adventure...." What does she have to lose? So of course she takes the chance, trusts her positive instincts, and she and her handsome prince live happily ever after.

This space is provided for your personal and/or support group notes.
PLEASE immediately record your ideas, insights, and inspirations as they occur to you.

11

The Cancer Conqueror suggests that our job is to become frog-kissers! Frog kissing is about love. "If I could give you just one piece of advice on how to conquer cancer, it would be to love, to be a frog-kisser. Nonjudgmental, unconditional love conquers cancer! And my advice would be to love yourself first—to kiss the frog in the mirror.... Healing has at its roots the ability to both give and receive nonjudgmental, unconditional love."

The 22 Non-Negotiable Laws of Wellness

In addition to the very powerful Law of Forgiveness that was illustrated by Greg's personal story of healing, there are many other profound truths to be found in this book. It is filled with inspiring stories of people whose lives have been enriched by adopting the practices and beliefs that Greg outlines.

One of the most surprising is the Law of Stress Hardiness; it is worth considering because we all have varying amounts of stress to deal with in our lives, sometimes vast amounts of it. Greg suggests that stress is not only to be expected but actually preferred:

> *We can and should develop a positive, workable approach to stress management.... Think of it. The perfect no-stress environment is the grave.... The problem isn't stress, it's toxic stress.... When we change our perception we gain control. The stress becomes a challenge, not a threat. When we commit to action, to actually doing something rather than feeling trapped by events, the stress in our life becomes manageable.*

Sometimes we can all use reminders for how we should be living—to keep our ideals foremost in our hearts and minds. Here are Greg's suggestions for resolving toxic stress and developing high self-esteem in the process:

11

- *REFRAME stress as a challenge and an opportunity for growth.*

- *INTERRUPT your cycles of fear, anger and guilt, and the build-up of stress and tension in your body.*

- *LEARN AND APPLY the simple but profound Serenity Prayer:*
    God, grant me the serenity
    To accept the things I cannot change,
    Courage to change the things I can,
    And the wisdom to know the difference.

This space is provided for your personal and/or support group notes.
PLEASE immediately record your ideas, insights, and inspirations as they occur to you.

11

- *QUIET AND ATTUNE your body-mind-spirit organism daily:*

    Step 1: Find a place where you can minimize distractions for a few minutes.

    Step 2: Sit quietly in a comfortable position.

    Step 3: Close your eyes; relax your muscles.

    Step 4: Breathe slowly and naturally. Silently repeat a focus word: "peace."

    Step 5: Keep your attention on your breathing and the focus word. When other thoughts come to mind say, "Oh well," and return to the repetition.

    Step 6: Continue for 10-20 minutes, once or twice per day. You are positively changing your very physiology with this practice.

- *ALLOW your playfulness to operate, especially in circumstances where you are likely to tense up.*

- *CHALLENGE irrational beliefs:*

    "My worth is dependent on never making mistakes."

    "My worth is dependent on being approved by others."

- *SUBSTITUTE more objective beliefs:*

    "Yes, I goofed. I make occasional mistakes like everyone."

    "Approval is nice but I did the right thing. I feel good about that."

- *GROW beyond a victim of circumstances to a master proactive creator of circumstances.*

11

There are other excellent books by Greg, including *Cancer: 50 Essential Things to Do* and *The Triumphant Patient*. These are invaluable resources for anyone dealing with cancer—or for those who want to find the motivation to make positive changes in their lives.

This space is provided for your personal and/or support group notes.
PLEASE immediately record your ideas, insights, and inspirations as they occur to you.

11

The Cancer Conqueror's Companion Ten Key Beliefs

The following beliefs are explained fully and are available in a brochure sent to cancer patients who contact CRFA. These understandings are based on what Greg discovered in his own healing journey, as well as what was consistently revealed in his scientific research on six hundred long-term survivors.

"There are moments when you are frightened, when it seems cancer may be getting the upper hand, when it seems all hope is gone. These thoughts were written for those moments. Can the human mind and spirit really affect the body? Certainly. After I was diagnosed with lung cancer and given 30 days to live, I went in search of cancer patients who had lived when they were supposed to die. Here, in summary, are the core survival beliefs I found. Use them.

"You, too, can conquer cancer!"

I Believe...

1) *I am in charge of my cancer, my cancer is not in charge of me.*

2) *Cancer is a reversible disease!*

3) *My treatment is effective and has minimal side effects.*

4) *My immune system is powerful.*

5) *My body, and thus my immune system, is affected by my mind and by my spirit.*

6) *My mind and my spirit are affected by my emotions.*

7) *Cancer is a message to change.*

8) *Peace is the goal.*

9) *Genuine peace comes from understanding there is a God who knows me and loves me. And God loves me even though God knows me.*

10) *I believe I become a Cancer Conqueror not because I go into remission, but because I become a new person!*

This space is provided for your personal and/or support group notes.
PLEASE immediately record your ideas, insights, and inspirations as they occur to you.

11

There is nothing like the sudden realization that our life may soon end to focus our mind and heart on important personal issues. Many people have put their lives on hold emotionally with respect to family, loved ones, and former relationships. From this perspective, the diagnosis of cancer can be seen as a kind of gift. It brings people together to share the burden of fighting against a life-threatening disease, but more importantly, to resolve any unfinished business in the process. What a shame that most of us bury these issues until the end looms in sight.

But do you really want to leave the moment of reconciliation and healing to the very end? That is for the movies; we do not need that kind of drama in our lives! Why not contact anyone with whom you have unfinished business and try to resolve issues now? That way, however the fight against your cancer turns out, you can experience the remainder of your life in peace. And maybe kiss a few more frogs along the way!

[Note from Cynthia: Greg was one of the first exceptional cancer survivors I asked to become a member of my Education Advisory Committee at the National Foundation for Alternative Medicine (NFAM). He had so much to teach other cancer patients. Greg's extraordinary and powerful personal story illustrates the ability of forgiveness and emotional release to reverse the course of terminal lung cancer. His recovery story was the most compelling I have ever heard and it forever changed my understanding of how people heal.]

Greg considers his release of anger and the extremely difficult but sincere act of forgiveness toward a former business associate to be the pivotal turning point in his illness. Based on what happened with his disease immediately following their encounter, this conclusion would appear to be irrefutable.

11

In 1984 Greg's doctors told him that he had about thirty days to live. Within a year, he made the decision to help others heal their cancer based on what he had learned through his own difficult journey. He founded the Cancer Recovery Foundation of America in 1985, which is now one of America's largest holistic cancer nonprofit organizations.

This space is provided for your personal and/or support group notes.
PLEASE immediately record your ideas, insights, and inspirations as they occur to you.

11

Contact Information

The Cancer Recovery Foundation
PO Box 238, Hershey, PA 17033
Phone: 800-238-6479
Fax: 717-545-7602
Website: www.cancerrecovery.org

[Note: The Cancer Recovery Foundation will schedule a free phone consultation to review your treatment options with you—whether you wish to discuss conventional, complementary, or alternative choices. First call them to request a packet of information to review.]

11

This space is provided for your personal and/or support group notes.
PLEASE immediately record your ideas, insights, and inspirations as they occur to you.

12

Part II

**Patient Action Plan
&
Resource Directory**

CHAPTER 12

A Formula for Healing

The new paradigm of (w)holistic medicine means treating the "whole" person, not just the physical body. It assumes the value of self-healing, demands a partnership between doctor/practitioner and patient, and recognizes the need to examine all aspects of an individual's life.

The body's innate wisdom and ability to heal itself surpass that of the most advanced medical technology, ancient herbal formula, or latest scientific breakthrough. To support these intrinsic healing abilities, consider the following five components of a holistic and comprehensive cancer treatment program. They speak to the understanding that the body is a self-cleansing, self-healing organism when it is given the proper tools. These five components (tools) must be considered, whether in a comprehensive general wellness or disease prevention program, or in a treatment protocol for advanced cancer.

Being in a state of optimal health and wellness normally involves harmony on all of these levels. If one is out of balance, less than optimal health and healing will usually ultimately result. Individuals should assemble a healthcare team in whom they have confidence to offer guidance about the most appropriate personal choices in the following categories:

1) The Psychological Aspects of Mental-Emotional Wellness and Balance, a Positive Attitude, and an Understanding of Life Purpose

   This is the most important component and the critical foundation of a comprehensive recovery plan. Because of this, it is the area that we have chosen to focus on most powerfully within this Report. Balance and strength in this area underlie the drive and determination to take on all the rest that, in most cases, needs to be embraced in order to heal. Identifying and releasing deep-seated (and many times unconscious) negative emotions and thought patterns, while maintaining an attitude of hope and positive beliefs, can make the all-important difference between healing and dying! It may sound simple, but it is not always easy.

12

233

This space is provided for your personal and/or support group notes.
PLEASE immediately record your ideas, insights, and inspirations as they occur to you.

12

Identifying emotional issues and the vitally necessary release work is probably the most dreaded, denied, and avoided part of any healing protocol. Our egos will convince us that we are okay, that we have either dealt with this area of our lives, or that any problems that exist are due to someone else's actions or attitudes. Sometimes we allow ourselves to experience, far too long, unexpressed anger, resentments, and/or unresolved grief over losses and other negative emotions and attitudes. When that happens, it often takes the body's development of cancer to jolt us into an awareness that we must make changes and deal with these issues. Finding out that you have cancer puts the need "to get right with your life," directly in your face. When there is nothing left to lose, the courage to address negative emotions and patterns of self-sabotage becomes easier to access and embrace.

For those who make the commitment to take on the challenging emotional and mental healing required, the life that emerges, in addition to being healthier, can be miraculously free and joyful. Survivors understand that the resulting changes and life-in-balance that emerge are vastly improved over what existed before. This is why we often hear from survivors that getting cancer, ironically, was the best thing that ever happened to them.

2) Detoxification

Because we live in an increasingly toxic world, the elimination and detoxification systems of the body must be strengthened. A highly toxic body cannot absorb the healthiest food and best supplements available because its systems do not function optimally and assimilation is compromised. As treatment protocols break down tumors in the body, it is critical that the body be able to quickly and efficiently eliminate the toxic by-products of these processes. Cancer patients are generally toxic to begin with. The number of cancers with a contributing factor of environmental toxicity is also a growing concern.

3) Nutrition, Diet, and Supplementation

In the alternative medicine world, it is typically accepted that an alkaline-based organic diet is optimal for the healing of cancer. There is a plethora of choices for supplementation. Most cancer patients do not die directly from their tumors; they die of malnutrition, toxemia, and/or

This space is provided for your personal and/or support group notes.
PLEASE immediately record your ideas, insights, and inspirations as they occur to you.

12

opportunistic infections. There are many advantages of introducing nutritional support for the diagnosed cancer patient. They include: avoidance of malnutrition, minimizing the side effects of toxic therapies, protecting healthy tissue, stimulating immune response, balancing hormones, modulating tumor growth factors, promoting healthy cell proliferation, increasing longevity, and improving quality of life.

4) Removal of Energy Blockages Throughout the Nervous System

As long as the physiological and mental/emotional aspects of homeostasis are recognized and addressed, the human organism can heal—this is our nature. Therapies can include chiropractic, acupuncture, bodywork, energy therapies such as Reiki and healing touch, sound, color and frequency therapies, homeopathy, electromagnetic therapies, vibrational medicine, and many others.

5) An Optimally Functioning Immune System

The immune system can be strengthened and supported by using innovative and relatively inexpensive natural methods and supplements. Positive results in strengthening immune response utilizing guided imagery have been documented for years by such highly regarded cancer experts as Bernie Siegel, MD, and O. Carl Simonton, MD.

These five components can also be incorporated into an integrative treatment approach as complementary therapies to surgery, chemotherapy, and radiation. Education and communication about these essential ingredients of a healthy life-style underlie the future of all effective disease treatments and preventions.

Because of the stories that we, the authors, have heard from cancer patients and cancer survivors over the years, and our own personal research, we have come to understand and believe that mental and emotional balance must be the foundation and keystone of any successful healing protocol. Without this balance, the rest of the treatments undertaken—no matter how advanced, innovative, and effective—are not built on solid ground. Although temporarily successful, they may not produce the long-term permanent recovery that is so desperately desired.

If you have cancer, we hope that this Report inspires you to listen to what your disease may be trying to tell you. Please seriously examine, with an open mind, the well-documented concepts we have presented, and fully realize that this is what a (w)holistic path of healing is really all about.

This space is provided for your personal and/or support group notes.
PLEASE immediately record your ideas, insights, and inspirations as they occur to you.

13

CHAPTER 13

Patients Personal Recovery Guide

We now reach across the time and space that separates us... to offer an impassioned plea that you hear what all these professionals are saying to you.

All of these researchers are telling you that if you are willing to do the work to identify your cancer-causing, unresolved emotional issues and eliminate them, you can achieve a complete and permanent recovery from most cancers.

Thanks in large part to Susan Silberstein and her experience of counseling over 25,000 cancer patients, this section of the Report contains your state-of-the-art, unique, one-of-a-kind Patients Personal Recovery Guide. This outstanding Guide will take you by the hand and help you to understand and identify your choices, and then decide what to do... step by step, to recover from cancer permanently.

This Patients Personal Recovery Guide is followed by what we believe to be the most extensive, comprehensive listing of patient resources in the world. Whatever your choices and needs are, you will find the help you require within this Comprehensive Support & Resource Directory.

A permanent recovery is our hope for each and every one of you. The truth about the potential causes and the potential cures of most cancers has been carefully gathered... these facts have been presented to you for your consideration.

You can do it... so many have now shown you the way....
Now you must take action....

We have designed this Patients Personal Recovery Guide to assist all who have psychologically induced cancer, fear its return, or wish to prevent ever getting it in the first place.

No matter who you are, the recovery plan and assistance you need are contained

This space is provided for your personal and/or support group notes.
PLEASE immediately record your ideas, insights, and inspirations as they occur to you.

13

in the balance of this Report.

For some, it will be a simple personal process at home, while others will need more help and/or a visit to one of the health centers described in this Report.

How simple can it be? Dr. Hamer perhaps says it best: "When the patient identifies the associated psychoemotional conflict and resolves it, the cancer will stop growing at the cellular level immediately... and the diseased tissue comes to be replaced by normal tissue."

Is it possible for you to do this now? Only you can answer this question. Many people have, and there are some wonderful success stories in this Report. You may wish to review the entire Dr. Hamer chapter and/or Greg Anderson's amazing recovery after being told he had only thirty days to live. Some of you will be able to emulate Greg's procedures and subsequently create your own recovery in a matter of days... as he did.

Some will need to seek out the help of a skilled therapist to discover and remove the cause of their cancer. Some of you will need a more detailed step-by-step approach.

But please be clear—regardless of your background or condition, the action plan and assistance you need to make informed decisions are presented in this Patients Personal Recovery Guide and the subsequent Comprehensive Support & Resource Directory.

Crucial Steps for Moving from Cancer Victim to Cancer Victor

By Susan Silberstein
Executive Director, Center for Advancement in Cancer Education

13

If you have been newly diagnosed with cancer, or have just been informed of a cancer recurrence, know that you have unlimited potential for self-help. You may wish to enlist the help of healthcare professionals as "coaches," or family and friends as "players" on your team, but ultimately you are the quarterback or captain: it is up to you to take control. Taking control not only empowers

This space is provided for your personal and/or support group notes.
PLEASE immediately record your ideas, insights, and inspirations as they occur to you.

13

you mentally; it also empowers your immune system. Now, how do you get started?

LESSON ONE: CREATE YOUR ACTION PLAN

Step #1: First, think about the following questions. The Center for Advancement in Cancer Education uses them as intake questions to help determine how the Center can best assist the cancer patients who seek it out. Then write down your answers to as many of the questions as possible. This will help you uncover where your immediate and long-term needs lie and will give you a starting point for assembling your "Healing Team" and creating your action plan.

Those patients who are most open and willing to dialogue on all of these issues place their Healing Team in the best position to be of real help. And those patients who manage to achieve a balance between cognition, emotion, and behavior are the most likely to outlive their prognosis with quality longevity.

[Space is provided to write down your answers to each question. Be realistic and answer them all as honestly as possible. This is a major part of your healing process.]

1) If treatment is now being administered, what kind is it, how do you feel about it and why?

_____

_____

_____

_____

_____

_____

_____

_____

13

This space is provided for your personal and/or support group notes.
PLEASE immediately record your ideas, insights, and inspirations as they occur to you.

13

2) Is any other treatment being considered? What has your doctor or health-care practitioner told you about this treatment, its risks, its benefits, its purpose, and expectations for outcome? How do you feel about this proposed treatment and why?

_____

_____

_____

_____

_____

_____

_____

_____

_____

_____

3) Are you seeking adjunctive/complementary support or a strictly alternative approach? Do you know what type or are you looking for options? Do you wish to learn more about any particular approaches?

_____

_____

_____

_____

_____

_____

_____

_____

_____

13

This space is provided for your personal and/or support group notes.
PLEASE immediately record your ideas, insights, and inspirations as they occur to you.

13

4) Do you need help deciding what type of healthcare professional to use? Do you need a referral?

_____

_____

_____

_____

_____

_____

_____

_____

_____

_____

_____

5) What are your financial limitations? What kind of insurance coverage do you have? What resources can you draw upon for treatments your insurance will not cover? (See chapter 14, your Comprehensive Support & Resource Directory)

_____

_____

_____

_____

_____

_____

_____

_____

_____

_____

13

This space is provided for your personal and/or support group notes.
PLEASE immediately record your ideas, insights, and inspirations as they occur to you.

13

6) What are your geographic limitations? How mobile are you?

_____

_____

_____

_____

_____

_____

_____

_____

_____

_____

7) How is your quality of life and how would you like to see this improve?

_____

_____

_____

_____

_____

_____

_____

_____

_____

_____

_____

13

This space is provided for your personal and/or support group notes.
PLEASE immediately record your ideas, insights, and inspirations as they occur to you.

13

8) What are your work commitments or other responsibilities and how flexible can you make these?

_____

_____

_____

_____

_____

_____

_____

_____

_____

_____

9) What is your family situation? Who else can be part of your support system? Would you like to find more support, and if so, from what type of source?

_____

_____

_____

_____

_____

_____

_____

_____

_____

_____

_____

_____

13

This space is provided for your personal and/or support group notes.
PLEASE immediately record your ideas, insights, and inspirations as they occur to you.

13

10) What were your eating patterns prior to diagnosis? To what extent have you changed these? To what extent are you willing to change these? What is your height/weight ratio? Who can help you shop for and prepare your food?

_____

_____

_____

_____

_____

_____

_____

_____

_____

_____

_____

11) How efficient are your digestion and elimination systems and would you like to learn more about improving these?

_____

_____

_____

_____

_____

_____

_____

_____

_____

_____

13

This space is provided for your personal and/or support group notes.
PLEASE immediately record your ideas, insights, and inspirations as they occur to you.

13

12) IMPORTANT: What stress patterns were present prior to being diagnosed? Which of these are not fully resolved?

_____

_____

_____

_____

_____

_____

_____

_____

_____

_____

_____

_____

13) What are your current stressors? Would you like help managing these?

_____

_____

_____

_____

_____

_____

_____

_____

_____

13

_____

_____

_____

This space is provided for your personal and/or support group notes.
PLEASE immediately record your ideas, insights, and inspirations as they occur to you.

13

14) IMPORTANT: Do you have any idea why you might have developed this cancer? What were your risk factors? Were there emotional factors, unresolved traumas, people, or situations to forgive and/or release? Could any life-style factors like smoking, alcohol, drugs, diet, work, or stress have played a role? Which of these factors are still operative in your life?

_____

_____

_____

_____

_____

_____

_____

_____

_____

_____

Those who have recovered, despite overwhelming odds, will tell you that they experienced some kind of paradigm shift in both attitude and life-style, that their recovery involved much more than just removal of symptoms, and that healing had to take place on multiple levels—physical, mental, emotional, and spiritual.

Step #2: Assemble your team—players and coaches—to the extent that you wish to have, and are able to identify, people who can help. Some positions may never get filled. You may need to interview several candidates for the positions and you may need to "hire" and "fire" periodically. Fill in their names in the space provided on the next page.

13

This space is provided for your personal and/or support group notes.
PLEASE immediately record your ideas, insights, and inspirations as they occur to you.

13

SUGGESTED TEAM MEMBERS

Research Director: Checks out resources on the internet and from cancer information centers.
Name_____Phone #_____

Head Librarian: Collects learning materials such as books, tapes, and reports.
Name_____Phone #_____

Director of Catering: Plans menus, reviews recipes, shops for food and prepares meals.
Name_____Phone #_____

Entertainment Chairperson: Compiles lists of and resources for activities that you consider "fun" (see below) and helps to facilitate your choices on a daily basis.
Name_____Phone #_____

Personal Trainer/Exercise Buddy: Keeps you on schedule with aerobic exercise routines, walking, yoga, tai chi, qi gong, etc.
Name_____Phone #_____

Spiritual Leader: Helps you with prayer and meditation. Remember the spirit dies before the body; to get well, you must engage your life force and spirit.
Name_____Phone #_____

Psychological Coach: Helps you change negative belief systems, provides emotional support, facilitates attitudinal healing, trains you in stress management, guides you with affirmations, and fosters your personal growth.
Name_____Phone #_____

Nutrition Coordinator: Tests for your biochemical individuality, prescribes herbs, enzymes, homeopathics, minerals, antioxidants, or other supplements.

13

This space is provided for your personal and/or support group notes.
PLEASE immediately record your ideas, insights, and inspirations as they occur to you.

13

Name_____Phone #_____

Detox Facilitator: Provides colon therapy, lymph drainage, or sauna; removes environmental toxins; trains you in other cleansing techniques.
Name_____Phone #_____

Medical Guide: Provides diagnostic and medical monitoring; presents treatment options; orders periodic tumor markers, immune profiles, hormone panels, and other, preferably non-invasive, tests. (See the "How to Choose a Holistic Practitioner" in the Resource Directory for this, as well as for sources for referrals.)
Name_____Phone #_____

Caution: Remember that all of these team members, helpers, liaisons, mentors, and guides must report back to you. They can help save you time and energy, facilitate your needs, handle important tasks, and provide valuable information, but you must still be the captain. They should only serve as your eyes, arms, and legs—never as your mind, heart, and "gut."

You will call upon them when needed, you will postpone their input when you are on "information overload," and you will filter their advice through your own intuitive knowing of what is right for you. Their job is not to shove down your throat, literally or figuratively, that which you cannot swallow. If they do not respect that, they should be replaced. If they really care about you, they will fully understand.

LESSON TWO: IDENTIFY YOUR NEEDS

The 12 most important questions to ask yourself are these:

1) Is tumor reduction immediately necessary? Is the tumor choking off vital life function like breathing, swallowing, or defecating? Is there intolerable pain?

_____

_____

_____

_____

13

This space is provided for your personal and/or support group notes.
PLEASE immediately record your ideas, insights, and inspirations as they occur to you.

13

Most cancer patients do not die of their tumors. They die of malnutrition, toxemia, and/or opportunistic infections. And they die of despair. Remember, healing is different from curing. Cure relates to removal of symptoms; healing relates to how you live your life. There are many cases in which the tumor may still be present, but the patient is vibrantly alive, and conversely, many cases in which the tumor is gone but the patient is dead.

2) If tumor reduction is not immediately necessary, am I ready to adopt a host-oriented approach in which the balanced function of every organ, system, and gland in my body becomes my goal?

_____

_____

_____

_____

_____

_____

This is hard work but do-able. Yet, you may recover, as many cancer patients have, simply by addressing only two basic issues: what you are eating and what is eating you.

3) Am I getting sufficient rest?

_____

_____

_____

_____

_____

_____

13

Cancer patients need a great deal of energy for healing. Many committed to recovery fail not because they do too little, but because they do too much. Avoid becoming a professional cancer patient 24/7. Remember to be a human BE-ing instead of a human DO-ing.

This space is provided for your personal and/or support group notes.
PLEASE immediately record your ideas, insights, and inspirations as they occur to you.

13

4) Am I eliminating what is toxic to my mind and body? Am I paying major attention to physical and emotional detoxification? Have I learned to detoxify my colon, lymph, liver, lungs, skin, and kidneys? Have I detoxified my mind and heart? Have I really eliminated all of my negative relationships (including those with people who have passed on)?

_____

_____

_____

_____

_____

_____

_____

_____

5) Have I learned to implement a healthy eating plan? Does my diet consist primarily of fresh, uncooked or lightly steamed plant foods like fruits, vegetables, seeds, and nuts, with a small amount of high-quality organic animal protein? Have I recognized that juicing is an excellent option to incorporate more fruits and vegetables in my diet?

_____

_____

_____

_____

_____

_____

_____

_____

13

This space is provided for your personal and/or support group notes.
PLEASE immediately record your ideas, insights, and inspirations as they occur to you.

13

6) Am I drinking half my weight or more in ounces of pure water daily? If not, why not?

_____

_____

_____

_____

_____

_____

_____

_____

_____

_____

_____

_____

7) Have I really learned to manage stress? Have I made a commitment to leave or change my stressful work environment? Have I learned which of my beliefs are health-promoting and which are disease-promoting? Have I learned to harness the former and change the latter?

_____

_____

_____

_____

_____

_____

_____

_____

_____

_____

13

This space is provided for your personal and/or support group notes.
PLEASE immediately record your ideas, insights, and inspirations as they occur to you.

13

8) Am I having fun?

_____

_____

_____

_____

_____

_____

_____

_____

_____

Fun heals. If life is not worth living, why bother? If you do not have a reason to get up in the morning, you might not. So compile a "Fun List"–a list of everything (simple or complex, plausible or implausible, easily attainable or seemingly impossible, important or frivolous, inexpensive or costly, time-consuming or of short duration) that could be considered FUN for you. Then every night before bed, pick one for tomorrow. It could be a creative hobby like basket weaving, plans for a major career change, a funny movie, a six-week getaway cruise, getting a puppy or going bowling. If you are not going to do this, please state why not.

_____

_____

_____

_____

_____

13

_____

_____

_____

_____

This space is provided for your personal and/or support group notes.
PLEASE immediately record your ideas, insights, and inspirations as they occur to you.

13

9) Do I follow a sensible aerobic exercise program?

_____

_____

_____

_____

_____

_____

_____

_____

_____

_____

Brisk walking, deep breathing, jumping rope, rebounding, dancing, gi gong, tai chi, or similar types of exercise bathe the body in essential oxygen, in the presence of which tumor cells cannot grow.

10) What message to change is my cancer sending me? An excellent exercise is to write yourself a letter from your disease, then answer it. Cancer is always a wake-up call to change something in our lives. What is it for me?

_____

_____

_____

_____

_____

_____

_____

_____

13

This space is provided for your personal and/or support group notes.
PLEASE immediately record your ideas, insights, and inspirations as they occur to you.

13

11) Have I mastered the Serenity Prayer?: "God grant me the serenity to accept the things I cannot change, the courage to change the things I can, and the wisdom to know the difference." You may wish to write this out on a 3 x 5 card, laminate it, and carry it with you at all times to read as many times as necessary during your day.

_____
_____
_____
_____
_____
_____
_____
_____
_____
_____

12) Do my reasons to live include helping others and being of service? Explain in detail how you will do this and/or who you intend to help.

_____
_____
_____
_____
_____
_____
_____
_____
_____
_____
_____
_____

13

This space is provided for your personal and/or support group notes.
PLEASE immediately record your ideas, insights, and inspirations as they occur to you.

13

LESSON THREE: PRIORITIZE YOUR NEEDS

Filling in a pie chart can help to show graphically the relative importance of your needs. For example, if you do a lot of exercise but have a terrible diet and are under a lot of stress, then the top priorities for you might be nutrition and stress management, represented by the largest slices of the pie. Your smallest slices may represent areas which are only slightly bothering you or which you would like to address at some point, if time and money permit, like hormone balance testing, pain management, or possible surgery. Very often, addressing the top priorities can also provide help with lesser priorities. For example, tumor reduction and pain management may actually be achieved with rest, nutrition, stress management, and detoxification.

Fun heals. If life is not worth living, why bother? If you do not have a reason to get up in the morning, you might not. So compile a "Fun List"–a list of everything (simple or complex, plausible or implausible, easily attainable or seemingly impossible, important or frivolous, inexpensive or costly, time-consuming or of short duration) that could be considered FUN for you. Then every night before bed, pick one for tomorrow. It could be a creative hobby like basket weaving, plans for a major career change, a funny movie, a six-week getaway cruise, getting a puppy or going bowling. If you are not going to do this, please state why not.

SAMPLE PIE CHART

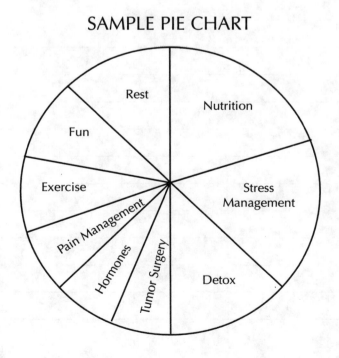

13

This space is provided for your personal and/or support group notes.
PLEASE immediately record your ideas, insights, and inspirations as they occur to you.

13

MY PIE CHART

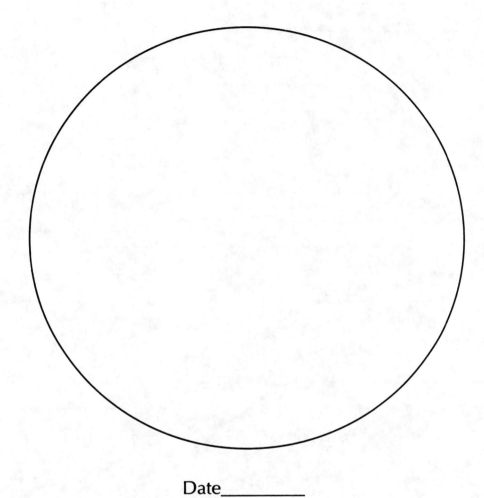

Date_____

We have provided several copies of this page, as your priorities may change over time and you will have to make revisions. Explain your current priorities below.

_____

_____

_____

_____

_____

_____

_____

13

This space is provided for your personal and/or support group notes.
PLEASE immediately record your ideas, insights, and inspirations as they occur to you.

13

MY PIE CHART

Date_____

Revised Priorities

_____

_____

_____

_____

_____

_____

_____

_____

13

This space is provided for your personal and/or support group notes.
PLEASE immediately record your ideas, insights, and inspirations as they occur to you.

13

MY PIE CHART

Date_____

Revised Priorities

_____

_____

_____

_____

_____

_____

_____

_____

13

This space is provided for your personal and/or support group notes.
PLEASE immediately record your ideas, insights, and inspirations as they occur to you.

13

MY PIE CHART

Date_____

Revised Priorities

_____

_____

_____

_____

_____

_____

_____

_____

13

This space is provided for your personal and/or support group notes.
PLEASE immediately record your ideas, insights, and inspirations as they occur to you.

13

LESSON FOUR: USE GREG ANDERSON'S FORGIVENESS PROCESS

Remember Greg Anderson's process for mastering forgiveness and the powerful and immediate effect it had on his terminal lung cancer? You may want to reread chapter 11. He described it as follows:

Become aware of the person toward whom you feel hostility, express active release from that hostility, and picture good things happening to him or her.

Whom do you still need to forgive? What resentments, anger, rage, jealousy, fear, sorrow or disappointment do you need to release from your life? Include yourself (we are often our own worst critics and judges, and guilt can cripple an immune system). Make more copies of this page and take some time to really think about this before completing it, if needed. You may want to go through this process every day until all situations requiring release in your life feel healed.

Name: _____

Release: _____

_____

Affirm: _____

_____

Name: _____

Release: _____

_____

Affirm: _____

_____

Name: _____

Release: _____

_____

Affirm: _____

_____

13

This space is provided for your personal and/or support group notes.
PLEASE immediately record your ideas, insights, and inspirations as they occur to you.

13

Name: _____
Release: _____

_____

Affirm: _____

_____

Name: _____
Release: _____

_____

Affirm: _____

_____

Name: _____
Release: _____

_____

Affirm: _____

_____

Name: _____
Release: _____

_____

Affirm: _____

_____

Name: _____
Release: _____

_____

Affirm: _____

_____

13

Name: _____
Release: _____

_____

Affirm: _____

_____

This space is provided for your personal and/or support group notes.
PLEASE immediately record your ideas, insights, and inspirations as they occur to you.

13

Name: _____
Release: _____

_____

Affirm: _____

_____

Name: _____
Release: _____

_____

Affirm: _____

_____

Name: _____
Release: _____

_____

Affirm: _____

_____

Name: _____
Release: _____

_____

Affirm: _____

_____

Name: _____
Release: _____

_____

Affirm: _____

_____

Name: _____
Release: _____

_____

Affirm: _____

_____

13

This space is provided for your personal and/or support group notes.
PLEASE immediately record your ideas, insights, and inspirations as they occur to you.

13

LESSON FIVE: CREATE YOUR PERSONAL GAME PLAN

The game plan consists of filling in your top goals, the specific priorities required to achieve those goals, the players/coaches on your team who will be helping, the specific task(s) to be done, and the study material that may be useful. The bad news is that you cannot do it all. The good news is that you probably will not have to.

SAMPLE GAME PLAN

[Note: This Sample Game Plan includes hypothetical player/coach names but the suggestions for the study materials are real people and guides.]

Goal #1: Nutrition

Priority #1: Eat healthier

Player/Coach #1: Husband Jim   Task: Shop at health store

Player/Coach #2: Sister Sue   Task: Cook dinner

Study Material: Patrick Quillan, author of *Beating Cancer With Nutrition*

Priority #2: Take nutritional supplements

Player/Coach #1: Dr. John   Task: Nutritional analysis/lab work

Study Material: Ann Wigmore, *The Wheatgrass Book*

Goal #2: Stress Management

Priority #1: Relaxation

Player/Coach #1: Dr. Barnes   Task: Hypnosis

Study Material: Lawrence LeShan, *Cancer As A Turning Point*

Priority #2: Yoga

Player/Coach #1: Yogi Anandra   Task: 2 Classes per week

Study Material: Yoga video

13

This space is provided for your personal and/or support group notes.
PLEASE immediately record your ideas, insights, and inspirations as they occur to you.

13

Goal #3: Detoxification

   Priority #1: Mercury elimination

      Player/Coach #1: Dr. Hudson   Task: Replace fillings

   Priority #2 : Drink Essiac tea

      Player/Coach #1: Sister Sue   Task: Pick up at health store

      Player/Coach #2: Husband Jim   Task: Brew tea daily

   Priority #3: Improve bowel function

      Player/Coach #1: Nurse Ratchett   Task: Weekly colonics

      Study Material: Bernard Jensen, *Colon Health*

Goal #4: Get more rest

   Priority #1: Outsource childcare

      Player/Coach #1: Neighbor Jan   Task: Pick up kids from soccer

   Priority #2: Cut back work hours

      Player/Coach #1: Me   Task: Talk to Kay at office

Goal #5: Do something just for myself

   Priority #1: Make appointment for a manicure

      Player/Coach #1: Husband Jim   Task: Take kids to a movie

Several sets of blank game plans are provided for you for use as your plan changes. Leave the last set of the "My Game Plan" worksheet pages blank in case you need more. Just photocopy additional sets as needed, as your game plan may shift frequently.

13

This space is provided for your personal and/or support group notes.
PLEASE immediately record your ideas, insights, and inspirations as they occur to you.

13

MY GAME PLAN—Date_____

Goal #1:_____

    Priority #1:_____

        Player/Coach #1:_____ Task:_____

        Player/Coach #2:_____ Task:_____

        Study Material:_____

    Priority #2:_____

        Player/Coach #1:_____ Task:_____

        Player/Coach #2:_____ Task:_____

        Study Material:_____

    Priority #3:_____

        Player/Coach #1:_____ Task:_____

        Player/Coach #2:_____ Task:_____

        Study Material:_____

Goal #2:_____

    Priority #1:_____

        Player/Coach #1:_____ Task:_____

        Player/Coach #2:_____ Task:_____

        Study Material:_____

    Priority #2:_____

        Player/Coach #1:_____ Task:_____

        Player/Coach #2:_____ Task:_____

        Study Material:_____

13

This space is provided for your personal and/or support group notes.
PLEASE immediately record your ideas, insights, and inspirations as they occur to you.

13

Goal #3:_____

  Priority #1:_____

    Player/Coach #1:_____ Task:_____

    Player/Coach #2:_____ Task:_____

    Study Material:_____

  Priority #2:_____

    Player/Coach #1:_____ Task:_____

    Player/Coach #2:_____ Task:_____

    Study Material:_____

Goal #4:_____

  Priority #1:_____

    Player/Coach #1:_____ Task:_____

    Player/Coach #2:_____ Task:_____

    Study Material:_____

  Priority #2:_____

    Player/Coach #1:_____ Task:_____

    Player/Coach #2:_____ Task:_____

    Study Material:_____

Goal #5:_____

  Priority #1:_____

    Player/Coach #1:_____ Task:_____

    Player/Coach #2:_____ Task:_____

    Study Material:_____

13

This space is provided for your personal and/or support group notes.
PLEASE immediately record your ideas, insights, and inspirations as they occur to you.

13

MY GAME PLAN—Date_____

Goal #1:_____

    Priority #1:_____

        Player/Coach #1:_____ Task:_____

        Player/Coach #2:_____ Task:_____

        Study Material:_____

    Priority #2:_____

        Player/Coach #1:_____ Task:_____

        Player/Coach #2:_____ Task:_____

        Study Material:_____

    Priority #3:_____

        Player/Coach #1:_____ Task:_____

        Player/Coach #2:_____ Task:_____

        Study Material:_____

Goal #2:_____

    Priority #1:_____

        Player/Coach #1:_____ Task:_____

        Player/Coach #2:_____ Task:_____

        Study Material:_____

    Priority #2:_____

        Player/Coach #1:_____ Task:_____

        Player/Coach #2:_____ Task:_____

        Study Material:_____

13

This space is provided for your personal and/or support group notes.
PLEASE immediately record your ideas, insights, and inspirations as they occur to you.

13

Goal #3:_____

    Priority #1:_____

        Player/Coach #1:_____ Task:_____

        Player/Coach #2:_____ Task:_____

        Study Material:_____

    Priority #2:_____

        Player/Coach #1:_____ Task:_____

        Player/Coach #2:_____ Task:_____

        Study Material:_____

Goal #4:_____

    Priority #1:_____

        Player/Coach #1:_____ Task:_____

        Player/Coach #2:_____ Task:_____

        Study Material:_____

    Priority #2:_____

        Player/Coach #1:_____ Task:_____

        Player/Coach #2:_____ Task:_____

        Study Material:_____

Goal #5:_____

    Priority #1:_____

        Player/Coach #1:_____ Task:_____

        Player/Coach #2:_____ Task:_____

        Study Material:_____

13

This space is provided for your personal and/or support group notes.
PLEASE immediately record your ideas, insights, and inspirations as they occur to you.

13

MY GAME PLAN—Date_____

Goal #1:_____

   Priority #1:_____

      Player/Coach #1:_____ Task:_____

      Player/Coach #2:_____ Task:_____

      Study Material:_____

   Priority #2:_____

      Player/Coach #1:_____ Task:_____

      Player/Coach #2:_____ Task:_____

      Study Material:_____

   Priority #3:_____

      Player/Coach #1:_____ Task:_____

      Player/Coach #2:_____ Task:_____

      Study Material:_____

Goal #2:_____

   Priority #1:_____

      Player/Coach #1:_____ Task:_____

      Player/Coach #2:_____ Task:_____

      Study Material:_____

   Priority #2:_____

      Player/Coach #1:_____ Task:_____

      Player/Coach #2:_____ Task:_____

      Study Material:_____

13

This space is provided for your personal and/or support group notes.
PLEASE immediately record your ideas, insights, and inspirations as they occur to you.

13

Goal #3:_____

    Priority #1:_____

        Player/Coach #1:_____ Task:_____

        Player/Coach #2:_____ Task:_____

        Study Material:_____

    Priority #2:_____

        Player/Coach #1:_____ Task:_____

        Player/Coach #2:_____ Task:_____

        Study Material:_____

Goal #4:_____

    Priority #1:_____

        Player/Coach #1:_____ Task:_____

        Player/Coach #2:_____ Task:_____

        Study Material:_____

    Priority #2:_____

        Player/Coach #1:_____ Task:_____

        Player/Coach #2:_____ Task:_____

        Study Material:_____

Goal #5:_____

    Priority #1:_____

        Player/Coach #1:_____ Task:_____

        Player/Coach #2:_____ Task:_____

        Study Material:_____

13

This space is provided for your personal and/or support group notes.
PLEASE immediately record your ideas, insights, and inspirations as they occur to you.

14

CHAPTER 14

Comprehensive Support
& Resource Directory

[Note from Cynthia: This is an eclectic list of helpful resources compiled from a variety of sources and the files that I helped create for the National Foundation for Alternative Medicine.]

Organizations that Specialize in
Alternative Medicine Information and Referrals

Cancer Report

John R. Voell and Cynthia A. Chatfield
PO Box 9211, Naples, FL 34101
Phone: 239-530-1376
Fax: 239-530-1375
Email: john@cancer-report.com or cynthia@cancer-report.com
Website: www.cancer-report.com

This website provides further information about the *Cancer Report*. Future updates and other helpful products and services will be available.

Center for Advancement in Cancer Education

Susan Silberstein, PhD, Executive Director
300 E. Lancaster Ave., Suite 100, Wynnewood, PA 19096
Phone: 610-642-4810
Fax: 610-896-6339
Email: caceinfo@comcast.net
Website: www.beatcancer.org

14

This space is provided for your personal and/or support group notes.
PLEASE immediately record your ideas, insights, and inspirations as they occur to you.

14

This is a non-profit cancer information, counseling, and referral agency that focuses on combining the body's natural healing potential with advances in medical science. The Center offers nutritional, immunological, and psychological resources for cancer prevention as well as non-toxic approaches as adjuncts or alternatives to conventional cancer treatments. This is a great resource and place to begin exploring options. Phone and in-person consultations by trained counselors are available. No fee. A donation is suggested.

The Moss Reports
Ralph W. Moss, PhD

PO Box 8183, State College, PA 16803
Phone: 800-980-1234 or 814-238-3369
Fax: 814-238-5865
Email: info@cancerdecisions.com
Websites: www.cancerdecisions.com and www.ralphmoss.com

Cancer researcher and author Ralph Moss creates individualized reports (currently priced at $297) recommending the best alternative and complementary treatments and clinics, including overseas, for specific types of cancer. Free information, an excellent weekly newsletter, and patient testimonials are also available at the website.

CANHELP, Inc.
Pat McGrady

32220 Rainier Avenue NE, PO Box 103, Port Gamble, WA 98364
Phone: 800-565-1732 or 360-297-5221
Fax: 360-297-6667
Email: canhelp@centurytel.net or madeleen@canhelp.com
Website: www.canhelp.com

CANHELP prepares detailed, individualized, professional reports to help cancer patients with their treatment options. Costs vary from $350-$450 depending on how quickly information is needed.

This space is provided for your personal and/or support group notes.
PLEASE immediately record your ideas, insights, and inspirations as they occur to you.

14

People Against Cancer

Frank Wiewal

604 East St., PO Box 10, Otho, IA 50569
Phone: 515-972-4444
FAX: 515-972-4415
Email: info@peopleagainstcancer.com
Website: www.peopleagainstcancer.com

A non-profit organization that offers personalized medical consulting services utilizing an international database of physicians and researchers at a membership cost of $500. Free information and newsletter.

People Against Cancer—Germany

Menschen Gegen Krebs, Cannstatter Str. 13, Kernen, Germany 71394
Phone: 49-715-191-0217 (add 011 to the beginning of this number if calling Germany direct from the U.S.)
Fax: 49-715-191-0218
Email: nexus@GMBH-Online.de or lothar@sensei.de
Website: www.krebstherapien.de

This is the European office for this cancer information, education, and referral organization. It uses the same personalized medical consulting protocol its American sister organization uses. English spoken.

German time is 6 hours ahead of U.S. Eastern time.

The National Foundation for Alternative Medicine (NFAM)

5 Thomas Circle NW, Suite 500, Washington, DC 20005
Phone: 202-463-4900
Email: inquire@nfam.org
Website: www.nfam.org

NFAM is a research organization and does not make personal recommendations or referrals. Information on the website changes periodically and may focus on diseases other than cancer. Founded by former U.S. Congressman, Berkley Bedell.

14

This space is provided for your personal and/or support group notes.
PLEASE immediately record your ideas, insights, and inspirations as they occur to you.

14

Legal, Financial, and Insurance Resources

General Suggestions for Financial Assistance:

Community voluntary agencies and service organizations such as the Salvation Army, Lutheran Social Services, Jewish Social Services, Catholic Charities, and the Lions Club may offer help. These organizations are listed in your local phone directory. Some churches and synagogues may provide financial help or services to their members.

Fundraising is another mechanism to consider. Some patients find that friends, family, and community members are willing to contribute financially if they are aware of a difficult situation. Contact your local library for information about how to organize fundraising efforts.

General Assistance programs provide food, housing, prescription drugs, and other medical expenses for those who are not eligible for other programs. Funds are often limited. Information can be obtained by contacting your state or local Department of Social Services; this number is found in the local telephone directory.

Corporate Angel Network

Phone: 914-328-1313
Email: info@corpangelnetwork.org
Website: www.corpangelnetwork.org

A non-profit organization that arranges and coordinates flights for cancer patients using the empty seats available on corporate aircraft.

National Patient Travel Center

Phone: 800-296-1217 (help line)
Website: www.patienttravel.org

Provides information about all forms of charitable, long-distance medical air transportation and provides referrals to all appropriate sources of help available in the national charitable medical air transportation network.

Call the Help Line that is staffed live 9AM to 5PM Eastern Time (Monday-

14

313

This space is provided for your personal and/or support group notes.
PLEASE immediately record your ideas, insights, and inspirations as they occur to you.

14

Friday). After hours help is available within 10 minutes of leaving an after-hours message marked "urgent."

Airlifeline

Phone: 877-AIR-LIFE (247-5433)
Website: www.airlifeline.org

A free nationwide service that flies qualified patients to treatment centers.

Angel Flight Central

Phone: 800-474-WING (9464) or 816-421-2300
Email: wings@angelflightcentral.org
Website: www.angelflightcentral.org

A non-profit organization dedicated to providing air transportation to those with special needs who demonstrate financial hardship. Serves 10 Midwestern states, see website for list.

The Center for Patient Advocacy

Phone: 800-846-7444
Website: www.patientadvocacy.org

Provides assistance to patients for navigating the managed care health system.

Patient Advocate Foundation

Phone: 800-532-5274
Website: www.patientadvocate.org

A national non-profit organization that serves as a liaison between patient and insurance company to resolve matters relating to diagnosis. Offers resources such as Patient Pal, a guide to help patients with insurance issues.

A Cancer Survivor's Almanac: Charting Your Journey

14

This reference book from the National Coalition for Cancer Survivorship includes thorough and easy to understand information about public and private health insurance, survivorship issues, disability benefits, employment rights, and legal and financial concerns. See next listing for order information.

This space is provided for your personal and/or support group notes.
PLEASE immediately record your ideas, insights, and inspirations as they occur to you.

14

What Cancer Survivors Need to Know About Health Insurance

For this publication and the previous one, contact:

National Coalition for Cancer Survivorship

1010 Wayne Avenue, Suite 770, Silver Spring, MD 20910
Phone: 301-650-9127 or (toll-free) 877-622-7937
Website: www.canceradvocacy.org

Provides information about health insurance and how to receive maximum reimbursement for claims.

Cancer Care, Inc.

Phone: 800-813-HOPE (4673)
Website: www.cancercare.org

A toll-free counseling line staffed with trained social workers who can suggest referrals for financial assistance.

The National Financial Resources Guidebook for Patients

Phone: 800-532-5274 (Patient Advocate Foundation)
Website: www.patientadvocate.org

Provides listings of Federal and State resources for obtaining financial assistance for a broad range of needs including housing, transportation, utilities, medical payments, and insurance deductibles.

NABCO Breast Cancer Resource List

Phone: 888-80-NABCO (806-2226)
Website: www.nabco.org (entire resource list)

Published by The National Alliance of Breast Cancer Organizations, this is an extensive (150 pages) and well-researched list of various resources for both cancer patients (much applies to ALL forms of cancer) and healthcare professionals. Contacts for treatment options, counseling, self-help, breast cancer support group listings and locations, advance directives, psycho-spiritual issues, information sources, risk/detection issues, financial/legal/insurance resources

14

This space is provided for your personal and/or support group notes.
PLEASE immediately record your ideas, insights, and inspirations as they occur to you.

14

(some are listed here as well), and much more. There is an extensive section on Spanish language resources.

National Association of Hospital Hospitality Houses

Phone: 800-542-9730
Website: www.nahhh.org

Lists more than 150 in U.S. that provide family-centered lodging and support services for patients receiving treatment far from home.

The Center for Medicare Advocacy, Inc.

Phone: 860-456-7790
Website: www.medicareadvocacy.org

A non-profit organization that provides education, advocacy, and legal assistance to help Medicare beneficiaries obtain necessary health care.

Medicaid (Medical Assistance)

Web site: www.hcfa.gov/medicaid/medicaid.htm

A jointly-funded Federal-State health insurance program for people who need financial assistance for medical expenses, coordinated by the Health Care Financing Administration (HCFA). At a minimum, states must provide home care services to people who receive Federal income assistance such as Social Security Income and Aid to Families with Dependent Children. Medicaid coverage includes part-time nursing, home care aide services, and medical supplies and equipment. Information about coverage is available from local state welfare offices, state health departments, state social services agencies or the state Medicaid office. Check the local telephone directory for the number to call. Information about specific state locations is also available on the HCFA website. Spanish-speaking staff is available in some offices.

14

This space is provided for your personal and/or support group notes.
PLEASE immediately record your ideas, insights, and inspirations as they occur to you.

14

Medicare

Phone: 800-MEDICAR (633-4227) TTY (for deaf and hard of hearing callers): 877-486-2048
Website: www.medicare.gov

This is a Federal health insurance program also administered by HCFA. Eligible individuals include those who are sixty-five or older, people of any age with permanent kidney failure, and disabled people under age 65. Medicare may offer reimbursement for some home care services. Cancer patients who qualify for Medicare may also be eligible for coverage of hospice services if they are accepted into a Medicare-certified hospice program. To receive information on eligibility, explanations of coverage, and related publications, call Medicare at the number listed above or visit their website. Some publications are available in Spanish.

Social Security Benefits or Supplemental Security Income (SSI)

Phone: 800-772-1213
Website: www.ssa.gov

You may be eligible for these and also food stamps and Medicaid. Call the toll-free Social Security Administration number listed above or contact your local office. Social Security provides a monthly income for eligible elderly and disabled individuals. Information on eligibility, coverage, and how to apply for benefits is available from the Social Security Administration. Supplemental Security Income (SSI) supplements Social Security payments for individuals who have certain income and resource levels. SSI is administered by the Social Security Administration. Information on eligibility, coverage, and how to file a claim is available from the Social Security Administration.

The State Children's Health Insurance Program (SCHIP)

Phone: 877-KIDS-NOW (543-7669)
Web site: www.insurekidsnow.gov

14

This is a Federal-State partnership that offers low-cost or free health insurance coverage to uninsured children of low-wage, working parents. Callers will be referred to the SCHIP program in their state for further information about what the program covers, who is eligible and the minimum qualifications.

This space is provided for your personal and/or support group notes.
PLEASE immediately record your ideas, insights, and inspirations as they occur to you.

14

Veterans Benefits

Phone: 800-827-1000
Website: www.va.gov/vbs

Eligible veterans and their dependents may receive cancer treatment at a Veterans Administration Medical Center. Treatment for service-connected conditions is provided and treatment for other conditions may be available based on the veteran's financial need. Some publications are available in Spanish. Spanish-speaking staff available in some offices.

State Departments of Insurance or State Departments of Health

Some states sell special health insurance for people with serious medical conditions who cannot find insurance elsewhere and who are "hard to insure." Contact your state office for more information.

The Hill-Burton Program

Phone: 800-638-0742
Website: www.hrsa.gov/osp/dfcr

This is a Federal program that requires participating hospitals and other facilities to provide a certain amount of free or reduced-fee care to those unable to pay. Not available at all hospitals and each hospital determines what is available.

Cancer Treatments Your Insurance Should Cover

Website: www.accc-cancer.org

Published by the Association of Community Cancer Centers, this brochure describes the minimum standard and investigational treatments that should be covered and what to do if reimbursement is denied.

The American Cancer Society (ACS)

Phone: 800-ACS-2345 (227-2345)
Website: www.cancer.org

This national office can provide the telephone number of the local ACS office

14

323

This space is provided for your personal and/or support group notes.
PLEASE immediately record your ideas, insights, and inspirations as they occur to you.

14

serving your area. The local ACS office may offer reimbursement for expenses related to cancer treatment including transportation, medicine, and medical supplies. The ACS also offers programs that help cancer patients, family members, and friends cope with the emotional challenges they face. Some publications are available in Spanish. Spanish-speaking staff available.

The AVONCares Program for Medically Underserved Women

Phone: 800-813-HOPE (4673)
Website: www.cancercare.org

Provides financial assistance and relevant education and support to low income, under-insured, and uninsured, underserved women throughout the country in need of diagnostic and/or related services (transportation, child care, and social support) for the treatment of breast, cervical, and ovarian cancers.

The Candlelighters Childhood Cancer Foundation (CCCF)

Phone: 800-366-CCCF (2223)
Website: www.candlelighters.org

CCCF is a non-profit organization that provides information, peer support, and advocacy through publications, an information clearinghouse, and a network of local support groups. CCCF maintains a list of organizations to which eligible families may apply for financial assistance.

Visionary Alternatives, Inc.

Phone: (toll-free) 866-750-4551
Website: www.visionaryalternatives.com

Provides some funding from alternative funding choices for patients with life-threatening illness who cannot afford this; also provides other suggestions for reduced costs for treatment.

14

This space is provided for your personal and/or support group notes.
PLEASE immediately record your ideas, insights, and inspirations as they occur to you.

14

The Leukemia and Lymphoma Society (LLS)

Phone: 800-955-4572
Website: www.leukemia-lymphoma.org

Offers information and financial aid to patients who have leukemia, non-Hodgkin's lymphoma, Hodgkin's disease, or multiple myeloma. Callers may request a booklet describing LLS's Patient Aid Program or the telephone number for their local LLS office. Some publications are available in Spanish.

SHARE

Phone: (toll-free) 866-891-2392
Website: www.sharecancersupport.org

A non-profit organization that provides support services for anyone affected by breast or ovarian cancer. SHARE's services include information hotline in English and Spanish, survivor-led support groups, public education, advocacy, and wellness programs. SHARE's model of survivorship also promotes public awareness and early detection of these diseases.

Alir

814 Highway A1A, Suite 302, Ponte Vedra Beach, FL 32082
Phone: (toll-free) 888-599-1112   Florida: 904-280-1112
Fax: 904-280-2010
Website: www.e-alir.com

This company offers a financial option for people who already own a life insurance policy. A life settlement allows an individual to turn an existing policy into an asset that can be used immediately. An investment company, called a funding or provider company, can purchase a life insurance policy from an individual. This provides the owner of the policy with a lump sum of cash (discounted from the face amount of the policy) and the end of premium payments. In return, the owner relinquishes all rights and future benefits from the policy. Online application available.

14

This space is provided for your personal and/or support group notes.
PLEASE immediately record your ideas, insights, and inspirations as they occur to you.

14

How to Find a Holistic or Alternative Physician

[Note: Most larger communities have a holistic/alternative publication of some kind, generally available at local health food stores, "new age" type stores, or large holistic centers/clinics. Practitioners advertise and are listed or featured in publications, so this is a good place to start your search for local options.]

American College for Advancement in Medicine (ACAM)

23121 Verdugo Drive, Suite 204, Laguna Hills, CA 92653
Website: www.acam.org

A not-for-profit medical society dedicated to educating physicians and other healthcare professionals on the latest findings and emerging procedures in preventive/nutritional medicine. ACAM represents more than 1,000 physicians in 30 countries and there is a searchable database available on their website.

American Holistic Medical Association (AHMA)

12101 Menaul Blvd., NE, Suite C, Albuquerque, NM 87112
Phone: 505-292-7788
Email: info@holisticmedicine.org
Website: www.holisticmedicine.org

AHMA has a Directory of members throughout the country and requests a payment of $15 to obtain a copy. There is also an online searchable referral database. For an AHMA Referral Directory, phone the number listed above or send a check or money order for $15 to the address above. State that you are requesting a copy of the AHMA Referral Directory and include clearly printed shipping information.

American Academy of Environmental Medicine

701 E. Kellogg, Suite 625, Wichita, KS 67207
Phone: 316-684-5500
Fax: 316-684-5709
Email: administrator@aaem.com
Website: www.aaem.com

14

This space is provided for your personal and/or support group notes.
PLEASE immediately record your ideas, insights, and inspirations as they occur to you.

14

A medical society that focuses on the prevention and treatment of disease and imbalances in the body resulting from environmental stressors and toxins. These can include both internal components (psychological, genetic, malnutrition, biological mechanisms, etc.) and external components (organic inhalants such as dusts, molds, pollens; chemicals; infectious organisms; radiation; toxins and pesticides; electro-magnetic fields, etc.). There is an online database of Academy members who have successfully completed the "Core Curriculum" (consisting of four instructional courses) searchable by state or country. Referrals can also be requested by emailing referral@aaem.com.

American Association of Naturopathic Physicians (AANP)

8201 Greensboro Drive, Suite 300, McLean, VA 22102
Phone: 703-610-9037
Websites: www.healthy.net/aanp/aanpsearch.htm (searchable database) and www.naturopathic.org

Founded in 1985, the American Association of Naturopathic Physicians is the national professional society representing naturopathic physicians who are licensed or eligible for licensing as primary care providers, following a four-year educational program (similar to a four-year medical degree). Naturopathic medicine blends centuries-old natural, non-toxic therapies with current advances in the study of health and human systems, covering all aspects of family health from prenatal to geriatric care. Naturopathic physicians are the family practitioners of the alternative medicine field, studying herbal medicine, homeopathy, nutrition, detoxification procedures, etc. Naturopathic medicine concentrates on whole-patient wellness. The medicine is tailored to the patient and emphasizes prevention and self-care. Naturopathic medicine attempts to find the underlying cause of the patient's condition rather than focusing on symptomatic treatment. Naturopathic physicians cooperate with all other branches of medical science referring patients to other practitioners for diagnosis or treatment when appropriate.

14

[Note: Not all practitioners who use the title of naturopath have attended a four-year degree program and some degrees in this field are available through distance learning certification programs. Be sure to ask what training your practitioner has obtained if this is important to you.]

This space is provided for your personal and/or support group notes.
PLEASE immediately record your ideas, insights, and inspirations as they occur to you.

14

How to Choose a Holistic Practitioner

[From the American Holistic Medical Association website: www.holisticmedicine.org]

Your first responsibility as a patient/client is to select a practitioner who will join your "team" to support you in obtaining and maintaining optimum health for your body, mind, emotions, and spirit. While most holistic practitioners use modalities that are currently labeled "alternative medicine," the interests and practices of our members vary widely. Thus, one person might work primarily with nutrition and herbs, while another might look mainly at the spiritual aspects of health and disease. Other areas of interest include spinal manipulation and bodywork, "energy medicine," mind-body medicine, acupuncture, and stress management. It is important to remember that there are many different definitions of holistic medicine. When choosing a practitioner, make sure that individual has the same type of philosophy and uses the treatment modalities you are seeking.

The following considerations are offered as a guide to help you find a practitioner with whom you are comfortable. Optimum health is more likely to be present when you work with someone who is supportive of your efforts to be in charge of your life. Some of the criteria may not apply to all situations.

1) Does this practitioner have health professional relationships with others How did you hear about this practitioner? A personal referral is often more powerful than a professional referral. What do friends and other professionals say about this person? How does he/she feel about second opinions or your interest in alternative healthcare therapies/treatments? What technical certifications, professional organizations or hospital affiliations does this practitioner have?

2) How do YOU respond to this practitioner's office and staff? This environment reveals his/her attitudes and beliefs. Do you feel comfortable and cared for when you call or visit the office? Does the ambiance enhance that comfort? Does the staff further your sense of well-being? Are educational handouts available in the office or waiting room? Is your appointment time honored or do you have to wait?

3) Do you feel like a valued person working as a partner with this practitioner?

14

This space is provided for your personal and/or support group notes.
PLEASE immediately record your ideas, insights, and inspirations as they occur to you.

14

Healing is enhanced by a healthy relationship between patient/client and practitioner. Do you feel this practitioner is there for you? Do you feel trust and confidence? Does he/she seem to care about you, take your medical history personally and show an interest in your family, life-style, and diet? Are you told about various treatment options? Do each of you recognize that you need the other? Is the practitioner accessible? Are you able to discuss the financial aspects of your care openly and comfortably? Positive answers to these questions are evidence of your rightful place as a co-creator of this healing partnership.

4) Is your personal dignity respected? Any examination or interaction should be respectful of your personal dignity.

5) Does this practitioner honor your anxieties and fears? Is this practitioner sensitive enough to place him/herself in your position regarding fears and anxieties about an illness or proposed treatment?

6) What is the state of this practitioner's health? Does he/she appear to have a healthy life-style? Signs of overweight, overwork, smoking or drinking may indicate that he/she does not take care of him/herself. You will probably do best with a team member who is just as committed to good health as you are. The Biblical statement, "Physician, heal thyself," is paramount in a health-filled relationship.

7) Are you allowed time between diagnosis and treatment? Does this practitioner allow you the time to collect the educational and personal resources that you need to make a well-informed decision?

8) Are you treated as if this is an important, ongoing relationship? Are you notified of test results within a reasonable period of time? Are follow-up visits scheduled after treatment? Is there discussion of future health goals and not just the immediate matter at hand?

14

9) Do you feel unconditionally accepted by this practitioner? Unconditional acceptance allows you to get well in your unique way. Do you feel that you are accepted no matter what develops, no matter what decisions you make? Can the practitioner approach your care with an open mind, rather than with a predetermined treatment plan?

This space is provided for your personal and/or support group notes.
PLEASE immediately record your ideas, insights, and inspirations as they occur to you.

14

10) Would the practitioner offer to a member of his/her own family the same carefully chosen advice that he/she has offered to you?

11) Would you send the person most dear to you to this practitioner? Do you feel unconditionally accepted by this practitioner? Do you have such a strong feeling of caring, confidence, and trust in this practitioner that you would send him/her, with no misgivings, the person who is dearest to you? If so, then you have found that special person to be on your health team.

Selecting a CAM Practitioner

[From the National Center for Complementary & Alternative Medicine/NIH website: http://nccam.nih.gov/health/practitioner/index.htm]

Selecting a health care practitioner—of conventional or complementary and alternative medicine (CAM)—is an important decision and can be key to ensuring that you are receiving the best health care. The National Center for Complementary and Alternative Medicine (NCCAM) at the National Institutes of Health (NIH) has developed a fact sheet to answer frequently asked questions about selecting a CAM practitioner, such as issues to consider when making your decision and important questions to ask the practitioner you select.

Great Books for Cancer Patients

Cancer: 50 Essential Things to Do
by Greg Anderson

Written by a lung cancer survivor who was once given 30 days to live, this book contains an excellent overview of the many components of an action plan for healing. Easy to read and understand—a great book for someone just diagnosed and beginning the cancer journey to overcome hopelessness or inertia.

The 22 Non-Negotiable Laws of Wellness
by Greg Anderson

Empowering book with a comprehensive, easy to follow, and concise description of what healing is truly about: that everything we think, say, feel, and do has a direct impact on our physical and emotional health—yet we overlook

14

This space is provided for your personal and/or support group notes.
PLEASE immediately record your ideas, insights, and inspirations as they occur to you.

14

this fundamental truth every day. Contains one of the best stories we have encountered concerning the powerful role of forgiveness in healing and wellness, and how the author experienced this as the pivotal turning point in overcoming his late-stage terminal cancer.

The Cancer Conqueror
by Greg Anderson

Another great book and modern-day parable. This is the story of one cancer patient's search for help and healing, and the teachers he met along the way. Simple and easy to read and great for newly diagnosed patients.

Only available from The Cancer Recovery Foundation at: 717-545-7600 or on the website: www.cancerrecovery.org

Cancer as a Turning Point: A Handbook for People with Cancer, Their Families and Health Professionals
by Lawrence LeShan, PhD

Written by a psychotherapist who has worked with cancer patients for over 50 years, this classic book written by the "father of mind-body therapy" demonstrates how psychological change, together with medical treatment, can mobilize a compromised immune system for healing.

Beating Cancer with Nutrition
by Patrick Quillin, PhD

There is a new and revised edition with a great deal of excellent information and research on nutrition, detoxification, healing diet, and supplementation. Written in a very readable style by the Director of Nutrition for Cancer Treatment Centers of America. Includes a CD.

Love, Medicine & Miracles
by Bernie Siegel, MD

Lessons learned about self-healing from exceptional cancer survivors by this well-known surgeon turned mind/body/spirit healer and teacher. Unconditional love is the most powerful stimulant of the immune system. The truth is: love heals. Miracles happen to exceptional patients every day—patients who have the courage to love and those who have the courage to work with

14

This space is provided for your personal and/or support group notes.
PLEASE immediately record your ideas, insights, and inspirations as they occur to you.

14

their doctors to participate in and influence their own recovery. There are many other great works from Bernie (all highly recommended) including <u>Humor and Healing</u> and an audiotape: "Meditations for Enhancing Your Immune System: Strengthen Your Body's Ability to Heal."

The Definitive Guide to Cancer
by Burton Goldberg

Offers an overview of the specific cancer treatment protocols of 23 alternative physicians and other practitioners, as well as detailed explanations of many of the modalities used. A good place to start learning about alternative cancer treatments in clinical practice. One chapter is devoted to Dr. Douglas Brodie's protocol.

Anatomy of an Illness
by Norman Cousins

A short book and fast read. This is the man who taught us about the value of laughter and humor in healing, but this book is much more. It will make you think about the role your thoughts, attitudes, and emotions play in your health and ultimate well-being.

Quantum Healing: Exploring the Boundaries of Mind-Body Medicine
by Deepak Chopra, MD

Chopra asks an interesting question: Why, when your body mends a broken arm, is it not considered a miracle, but when your body rids itself of cancer, it is? Chopra believes the two phenomena spring from the same well, that the body is capable of doing much more than we assume it can. He calls this ability to cure disease from within "quantum healing," and shows how we are all capable of it. He believes intelligence exists everywhere in our bodies, in each of our 50 trillion cells, and that, therefore, each cell knows how to heal itself.

Healing Words: The Power of Prayer and the Practice of Medicine
by Larry Dossey, MD

This popular book studies the link between medicine and spirituality, and the healing power of prayer. Prayer heals? Hardly news in the religious world, but for modern science, it is a revelation, one confirmed by dozens of laboratory experiments that Dossey cites. Prayer can help with high blood pressure, asthma,

14

This space is provided for your personal and/or support group notes.
PLEASE immediately record your ideas, insights, and inspirations as they occur to you.

14

heart attacks, headaches, and anxiety; it can alter enzyme activity, blood cell growth, and even the germination of seeds. Another good read along these lines: Prayer Is Good Medicine, also by Dossey.

Molecules of Emotion: The Science Behind Mind-Body Medicine
by Candace Pert, PhD

The first book to scientifically explain and document exactly how our thoughts and emotions affect our physical health, and how the mind and body function together as parts of an interconnected system. Pert uses understandable terminology to explain the neuropeptide system as the carrier of the emotions throughout the entire body. Pert's discovery that neurotransmitters are found not only in the brain but also in the gut, the endocrine system, and the nervous system throughout the body, is the clearest proof to date that our emotions and thoughts have a direct and powerful effect on our health. Also by Dr. Pert: Your Body is Your Subconscious Mind: New Insights Into the Body/Mind Connection.

A General Theory of Love
by Thomas Lewis, MD, et. al.

New research in brain function by three psychiatrists has proven that love is a human necessity; its absence damages not only individuals, but also our whole society, and it explains how and why our brains have evolved to require consistent bonding and nurturing. The contributors contend that close emotional connections actually change neural patterns in those who engage in them, affecting our sense of self—convincingly connecting love and biology by discussing the hard facts behind the science of love.

The Type C Connection: The Behavioral Links to Cancer and Your Health
by Lydia Temoshok, PhD and Henry Dreher

In agreement with Dr. Douglas Brodie's empirical observations on the personality traits common to cancer patients, the authors describe the cancer-prone personality (Type "C") as those who typically have trouble expressing emotions; that deny anger or other negative emotions, and who generally try to help others at their own expense. The authors show how the immune system works. They describe how not shutting yourself down emotionally and

14

This space is provided for your personal and/or support group notes.
PLEASE immediately record your ideas, insights, and inspirations as they occur to you.

14

expressing your needs, anger, etc., can actually boost your immune system to fight cancer. An out-of-print book but you can find copies on Amazon.com and elsewhere.

Remarkable Recovery: What Extraordinary Healings Tell Us About Getting Well and Staying Well
by Caryle Hirshberg and Marc Ian Barasch

A compilation of scores of stories of spontaneous remission and other so-called anomalies in the recovery of terminal cancer patients. If you are looking for hope in the face of dire medical prognosis, here it is, documented by medical experts. Cases of patients who unexpectedly survive a terminal disease happen more often than is believed, and this book gives fully detailed histories of a number of long-term survivors. In fact, the authors show us that remarkable recoveries are much more than remissions and anything but spontaneous. They feel that these cases are clear demonstrations of the ability of the human body, mind, and spirit to heal itself.

Mind-Body Unity: A New Vision for Mind-Body Science and Medicine
by Henry Dreher

Over the past twenty years, an explosion of scientific studies has helped to explain why our emotional and mental states may exert such a strong influence on the state of our health. Dreher argues that our minds play a role in our health the way our eyes play a role in our sight. He discusses remarkable findings on the role of emotions, coping, and personality in cancer progression and survival. He describes mind-body approaches to the treatment of cancer and other health conditions.

The Creation of Health:
The Emotional, Psychological and Spiritual Responses That Promote Health and Healing
by Caroline Myss, PhD and C. Norman Shealy, MD

This is the unusual pairing of a well-known medical intuitive/theologian with a conventionally-trained neurosurgeon and past President of the American Holistic Medical Association. As a team that has worked with patients for many years, they explore the link between emotional dysfunction and physical illness; the emotional, physical, and spiritual patterns that form health; and the

14

This space is provided for your personal and/or support group notes.
PLEASE immediately record your ideas, insights, and inspirations as they occur to you.

14

stresses that can cause disease. There are discussions with case studies of specific diseases in terms of lifestyle factors, stress, psychological patterns, and energy factors. Other books by Caroline Myss: <u>Why People Don't Heal and How They Can</u> and <u>The Energetics of Healing</u>.

Heal Your Body: The Mental Causes for Physical Illness
by Louise Hay

An easy read, this book offers positive new thought patterns to replace negative emotions. It includes an alphabetical chart of physical ailments, the probable mental/emotional causes, and healing affirmations to help you eliminate old patterns. Louise Hay healed herself by using these techniques.

The Art of Forgiving: When You Need to Forgive and Don't Know How
by Lewis B. Smedes

"When we forgive," Smedes says, "we set a prisoner free and discover that the prisoner we set free is us." He teaches the reader that more than anything else, forgiveness is a way of healing. If you are ready to make peace with those who have hurt or betrayed you, then this practical book can be your roadmap. Dramatic examples from real life situations are used.

Living Well with Cancer
by Katen Moore, RN, AOCN, MSN and Libby Schmais, MFA

Written by an oncology nurse and medical researcher, this book addresses the side effects of medical treatments—from aches and pains to nausea, fatigue, fear, and depression, with down-to-earth recommendations. It addresses health-care issues rarely discussed in standard medical texts, including guidance on exercise, rest, nutrition, sex, and emotional issues. Includes a resource guide to helpful organizations and literature—lots of practical advice.

Hungry for Health
by Susan Silberstein, PhD

14

A practical lesson in healthful eating from the Executive Director of the Center for Advancement in Cancer Education. Great for anyone who wants to eat better, but does not know where to start or how to proceed. Based on four fundamental principles for preventing disease, enhancing wellness or facilitating healing.

This space is provided for your personal and/or support group notes.
PLEASE immediately record your ideas, insights, and inspirations as they occur to you.

14

Contains 157 no-guilt recipes with lots of tasty tips and "nutri-notes." Based on Dr. Silberstein's 28 years of experience with nutrition and cancer patients, although anyone who wants improved nutrition will benefit. Order online at www.beatcancer.org or call 610-642-4810.

Natural Compounds in Cancer Therapy
by John Boik

The ultimate reference book in understanding the use of natural botanical compounds in cancer therapy. A powerful starting point for cancer protocols involving vitamins, herbs, and other natural products.

Prescription for Nutritional Healing
by Phyllis Balch, CNC and James Balch, MD

This is the "bible" of reference books for nutritional guidance, organized by specific condition or disease, with an extensive list of recommended nutritional (drug-free) supplements, including vitamins, minerals, herbs, and other items. Includes scientific descriptions and uses of all supplements, as well as food recommendations, and other important considerations. Excellent resource to have on hand, and a great starting point to educate and inform. Updated regularly, current version is the third edition.

Be Prepared: The Complete Financial, Legal and Practical Guide for Living With a Life-Challenging Condition
by David S. Landay

Although not cancer-specific, this book offers excellent easy-to-understand and practical guidance.

VIDEOS/DVD's

Breast Cancer: The Diet Connection narrated by Susan Silberstein, PhD, Executive Director of the Center for the Advancement in Cancer Education.

The video outlines easy dietary steps to help prevent cancer or its recurrence; the information can be applied to all types of cancer, enhancing immune response and wellness. It is an excellent plan, based on Dr. Silberstein's 28 years of experience with over 25,000 cancer patients, and as many years studying and teaching proper nutrition. Includes references for research studies.

14

This space is provided for your personal and/or support group notes.
PLEASE immediately record your ideas, insights, and inspirations as they occur to you.

14

Kitchen Chemotherapy
by Susan Silberstein, PhD

Based on thousands of articles published in the scientific literature documenting the relationship between diet and cancer survival, this 79-minute CD highlights a dozen advantages of implementing nutrition in a cancer treatment program, outlines foods that promote or suppress tumor growth, and explains the connection between cancer and biological terrain.

Purchase online at www.beatcancer.org or call 610-642-4810.

What the Bleep Do We Know!?

This is a groundbreaking documentary/movie that is an entirely new type of film. It uses entertaining visual effects and story-telling to demonstrate the tenets of quantum physics and how they are actually the force behind the creation of our daily lives. Interviews with award winning physicists and other notable researchers and scientists, such as Candace Pert, are woven provocatively throughout the movie. If you would like to know more about the science behind how our thoughts and emotions create our reality, including our state of health, then you need to see this film!

See www.whatthebleep.com for more information or www.whatthebleep dvd.com for DVD ordering information.

Other Resources

Prepare For Surgery, Heal Faster

Created by psychotherapist Peggy Huddleston, this is a five-step program to release fear and mentally prepare for surgery in order to create the biochemistry of healing and speed recovery. Research on this program was conducted at a Harvard Medical School teaching hospital in Boston. Can also be used to lessen the side effects of chemotherapy, radiation or other invasive medical procedures. These workshops are now offered in hospitals, HMO's, and for individuals—by nurses and therapists trained and certified by Peggy.

Book and tape available on the website at www.healfaster.com or call 800-726-4173.

14

This space is provided for your personal and/or support group notes.
PLEASE immediately record your ideas, insights, and inspirations as they occur to you.

14

Writing About Cancer

A therapeutic writing course for cancer patients and survivors, created by professional writing teacher and author Margie Davis. There is an online therapeutic course offered three times a year, along with "Writing for Personal Caregivers." The work is based on the research by James D. Pennebaker, PhD, who found that exploring deep thoughts and feelings about stressful events through writing can help people heal, both emotionally and physically. Copies of Margie's therapeutic writing journal, The Healing Way, A Journal for Cancer Survivors, are available on her website. With over 60 writing exercises, this book encourages therapeutic writing at a cancer patient's own pace. Margie also licenses a four-week and a 2.5-hour "Writing About Cancer" program so facilitators may lead this program. For details go to www.writingtoheal.com.

Guided Imagery Programs

Although called "visualization" and "mental imagery," these terms can be misleading. Guided Imagery involves far more than just the visual sense—and this is a good thing, given the fact that only about 55% of the population is strongly wired visually. Instead, imagery involves all of the senses and almost anyone can do this. Neither is it strictly a "mental" activity—it involves the whole body, the emotions, and all the senses, and it is precisely this body-based focus that makes for its powerful impact.

Health Journeys

A private multimedia publishing company offering outstanding guided imagery CD's, tapes, and videos by Belleruth Naparstak, a gifted psychotherapist.

Cancer-related topics include "The Cancer Pack," "Chemotherapy, Anger & Forgiveness," "Healing Trauma," "Fight Cancer," and others. The music has been specially written in most "journeys" to synchronize perfectly with Belleruth's soothing voice. Additional products by other leaders in the mind-body field such as O. Carl Simonton, Bernie Siegel, and Andrew Weil are also available here. Great quality. There are free audio samples available online.

Website is www.healthjourneys.com or call 330-633-3831 or 800-800-8661.

14

This space is provided for your personal and/or support group notes.
PLEASE immediately record your ideas, insights, and inspirations as they occur to you.

14

Cancer Involvement Program

An integrative and holistic approach to cancer treatment, this program can be incorporated into a conventional or alternative treatment plan. Includes 9 guided imagery sessions (CD or cassettes), a manual called Understanding Your Journey, and an interactive journal/sketchbook. Guided Imagery sessions include visualizations for chemotherapy and radiation. They assist with depression, will to live, reducing tension and stress, facing fear, and enhancing the immune response.

Phone: (toll-free) 877-795-5824
Website: www.onehealthpublishing.com

Emotional Genius—How Your Emotions Can Save Your Life
by Karla McLaren

(Six 90-minute cassette tapes from www.soundstrue.com)

Without an understanding of our emotional nature, most people never succeed in their quest for health, happiness, and freedom. Our detachment from our true feelings is largely responsible for the lack of healthy relationships and the preponderance of disease. Karla teaches how to address disease by balancing the mind, body, spiritual, and emotional aspects of our being. The tapes contain exercises for addressing each of the emotions, including sadness, anger, and hate. Karla is an empath, teacher, and author who specializes in emotional trauma work. She states that roughly 50% of us are trauma survivors and teaches that all of our emotions, including the most difficult ones, are carriers of energy, information, and wisdom that have the power to protect and heal us. Although it does not replace the need for professional help, these tapes are a great self-help resource.

American Environmental Health Foundation
(For environmentally safe and non-toxic products)

14

A non-profit organization that personally reviews and approves most products offered in its catalog. Includes air purifiers, water filters, household cleaners, bath and bedding items, books and videos, lawn and garden supplies, paints and home improvement items, nutritional supplements, personal care items, saunas, and various pollution detection kits.

This space is provided for your personal and/or support group notes.
PLEASE immediately record your ideas, insights, and inspirations as they occur to you.

14

Phone: 800-428-2343 or fax catalog request to 214-361-2534
Email: aehf@aehf.com
Website: www.aehf.com (catalog is also online)

Internet Links for Additional Cancer and Alternative/Complementary Health Information

Government Websites

◆ www.nccam.nih.gov

Website for the National Center for Complementary and Alternative Medicine at the National Institutes of Health. For an excellent search engine on this site to find scientific and medical articles about specific treatments, go to CAM on PubMed at: www.nlm.nih.gov/nccam/camonpubmed.html.

◆ www.cancer.gov

Website for the National Cancer Institute with information about clinical trials and other related sites. CancerNet is a service of the National Cancer Institute and contains extensive resources for exploring more traditional treatment options, some alternative choices, and self-education. For the PDQ (Physicians Data Query) Clinic Trials Database, visit the NCI website: www.cancernet.nci.nih.gov or call 800-4-CANCER (422-6237) to search this comprehensive database of more than 1,800 active cancer trials.

◆ www.nlm.nih.gov/medlineplus/cancergeneral.html

NIH website for health information, cancer specific with links for the latest news in cancer treatments, both traditional and CAM.

Other Websites

◆ www.healingcancernaturally.com

14

A wealth of good information about mind-body healing, alternative methods, inspiration, downloads, and lots of links for more exploration. Includes articles about Dr. Hamer's work.

This space is provided for your personal and/or support group notes.
PLEASE immediately record your ideas, insights, and inspirations as they occur to you.

14

◆   www.annieappleseedproject.org

Extensive resources included. Site created by a breast cancer survivor. Includes a database of international clinics, environmental issues, multicultural issues, women's cancer issues, and more.

◆   www.heall.com/body/resource/organizations/cancer.html

An eclectic list of organizations and physicians who treat cancer world-wide. Both traditional and alternative medicine contact information is provided.

◆   www.gnc.com

GNC's (the vitamin store) website includes this excellent database (go to the "Health Notes" link) with descriptions of many health conditions, including which supplements have demonstrated benefits, with clinical efficacy ratings. Also includes listings for most vitamins, herbs, homeopathics, and other supplements with specific benefits, safety checker (drug/supplement interactions), and more. Great website for beginners to learn the basics about supplementation.

◆   www.healthy.net

HealthWorld website. Includes extensive wellness, nutrition, alternative medicine, and treatment information with healthcare provider referral networks available. Also links to MedLine searches at:
www.healthy.net/library/search/medline.asp

◆   www.cancerlinksusa.com

Links given to many cancer-related sites, including support groups, large cancer hospitals, and recent articles on cancer. There is an abbreviated glossary for many medical oncology terms at:
www.cancerlinksusa.com/tools/glossary.html

◆   www.cancer411.com

14

A great deal of information and resources about treating cancer, both traditionally and alternatively, with a good selection of additional sites to visit. Information about worldwide clinical trials listed.

This space is provided for your personal and/or support group notes.
PLEASE immediately record your ideas, insights, and inspirations as they occur to you.

14

- www.cancer.org

Website for the American Cancer Society. There is information about alternative and complementary options under "Treatment Options."

- www.crfa.org

If you are interested in clinical trials, there is an excellent explanation on the website of The Cancer Research Foundation of America designed to educate cancer patients about opportunities for becoming involved in cancer research studies and to help them make an informed decision about enrolling.

- www.mcphs.edu/MCPHSWeb/herbal

Website for the Longwood Herbal Task Force with scientific and research-based information about medicinal herbs and dietary supplements, including monographs, clinician information summaries, and patient fact sheets.

- www.herbmed.org

An interactive, electronic herbal database that offers hyperlinked access to the scientific data underlying the use of herbs for health—an evidence-based resource for professionals, researchers, and the public.

- www.ecap-online.org

Dr. Bernie Siegel's website for Exceptional Cancer Patients, the organization he founded in 1978 that promotes the concept of integrative healing in mind, body, and spirit. Offers professional training programs, as well as the Insights for Living Beyond Cancer program, and retreats for patients. Call 814-337-8192 or email: info@mind-body.org.

- www.5aday.com

Great website with free newsletter and a wealth of information about fruits and vegetables, includes lots of recipes.

- www.consumerlab.com

An independent lab that provides test results and information to help consumers and healthcare professionals evaluate health, wellness, and nutrition

14

products. It publishes results of its tests online and includes listings of brands that have passed testing. More than 1 in 5 products fail testing.

- www.gerson.org

Website for the Gerson Institute, with resources for exploring the Max Gerson juicing therapy. Includes case histories and survivor stories along with places to obtain the therapy or education.

- www.noah-health.org

This is the New York Online Access to Health page. You can search under a particular type of cancer, type of treatment or just "alternative treatment for cancer" with excellent results. There is information about prevention, risk factors, staging and grading of tumors, clinical trials, living with cancer, side effects and complications, some alternative and complementary therapies, additional information resources, and more.

- www.healthlobby.com

An advocacy website that lists states with favorable medical freedom laws for healthcare practitioners and offers updates on current legal agendas, alternative medicine political action, additional resources, etc. Find out which states currently have the most liberal "medical freedom" laws and where your state stands.

Cancer Report Order Form

Please send_____ copy(s) of the *Cancer Report* for $29.95 each or save 40% by getting a case of 11 for $197.67

Add S/H: 2-3 day delivery 1 Report $8.85 ◆7-10 day delivery 11 Reports $18.50

Check payment option below that applies to you.

__ Enclosed is a check or money order payable to:

Change Your World Press for $_____

__ Charge $_____ to credit card

Credit Card Information:

Visa - Master Card - Discover (circle one)

Card Number_____

Name as it appears on card: (please print clearly)

_____

Expiration Date_____

Signature (if not card holder)_____

Billing Address for Credit Card:

Name_____

Address_____

City_____ State____ Zip_____

Phone (include area code)_____

Email_____

for newsletter & updates. (Your email will not be sold or shared)

Ship Cancer Report(s) to:

Name_____

Address_____

City_____ State____ Zip_____

(If shipping outside the USA, please call or email for order information)

To Order:

Visit www.cancer-report.com

Or email order (with credit card information) to: ordernow@cancer-report.com

Or call: 239-530-1376 or fax order form to: 239-530-1375

Or mail order form and payment to:

Change Your World Press
PO Box 9211
Naples, FL 34101